# Nasal Airway Obstruction

*Editors*

JENNIFER A. VILLWOCK
RONALD B. KUPPERSMITH

# OTOLARYNGOLOGIC CLINICS OF NORTH AMERICA

www.oto.theclinics.com

*Consulting Editor*
SUJANA S. CHANDRASEKHAR

October 2018 • Volume 51 • Number 5

**ELSEVIER**

1600 John F. Kennedy Boulevard • Suite 1800 • Philadelphia, Pennsylvania, 19103-2899

http://www.oto.theclinics.com

**OTOLARYNGOLOGIC CLINICS OF NORTH AMERICA Volume 51, Number 5**
**October 2018 ISSN 0030-6665, ISBN-13: 978-0-323-64095-4**

Editor: Jessica McCool
Developmental Editor: Sara Watkins

*Otolaryngologic Clinics of North America* (ISSN 0030-6665) is published bimonthly by Elsevier, Inc., 360 Park Avenue South, New York, NY 10010-1710. Months of issue are February, April, June, August, October, and December. Business and Editorial Offices: 1600 John F. Kennedy Blvd., Suite 1800, Philadelphia, PA 19103-2899. Customer Service Office: 6277 Sea Harbor Drive, Orlando, FL 32887-4800. Periodicals postage paid at New York, NY and additional mailing offices. Subscription prices are $396.00 per year (US individuals), $835.00 per year (US institutions), $100.00 per year (US student/resident), $519.00 per year (Canadian individuals), $1058.00 per year (Canadian institutions), $556.00 per year (international individuals), $1058.00 per year (international institutions), $270.00 per year (international & Canadian student/resident). Foreign air speed delivery is included in all *Clinics'* subscription prices. All prices are subject to change without notice. **POSTMASTER:** Send address changes to *Otolaryngologic Clinics of North America*, Elsevier Health Sciences Division, Subscription Customer Service, 3251 Riverport Lane, Maryland Heights, MO 63043. **Telephone: 1-800-654-2452 (U.S. and Canada); 314-447-8871 (outside U.S. and Canada). Fax: 314-447-8029. E-mail: journalscustomerservice-usa@elsevier.com (for print support); journalsonlinesupport-usa@elsevier.com (for online support).**

*Reprints.* For copies of 100 or more of articles in this publication, please contact the Commercial Reprints Department, Elsevier Inc., 360 Park Avenue South, New York, NY 10010-1710. Tel.: 212-633-3874; Fax: 212-633-3820; E-mail: reprints@elsevier.com.

*Otolaryngologic Clinics of North America* is also published in Spanish by McGraw-Hill Interamericana Editores S.A., P.O. Box 5-237, 06500 Mexico D.F., Mexico.

*Otolaryngologic Clinics of North America* is covered in *MEDLINE/PubMed (Index Medicus), Current Contents/Clinical Medicine, Excerpta Medica, BIOSIS, Science Citation Index,* and *ISI/BIOMED.*

## PROGRAM OBJECTIVE

The goal of the *Otolaryngologic Clinics of North America* is to provide information on the latest trends in patient management, the newest advances; and provide a sound basis for choosing treatment options in the field of otolaryngology.

## LEARNING OBJECTIVES

Upon completion of this activity, participants will be able to:
1. Review diagnostic algorithm for evaluation of and medical treatment for nasal airway obstruction
2. Discuss surgical management of nasal valve collapse and non-allergic rhinitis.
3. Recognize nasal obstruction considerations in cosmetic rhinoplasty and sleep apnea.

## ACCREDITATION

The Elsevier Office of Continuing Medical Education (EOCME) is accredited by the Accreditation Council for Continuing Medical Education (ACCME) to provide continuing medical education for physicians.

The EOCME designates this enduring material for a maximum of 15 *AMA PRA Category 1 Credit*(s)™. Physicians should claim only the credit commensurate with the extent of their participation in the activity.

All other health care professionals requesting continuing education credit for this enduring material will be issued a certificate of participation.

## DISCLOSURE OF CONFLICTS OF INTEREST

The EOCME assesses conflict of interest with its instructors, faculty, planners, and other individuals who are in a position to control the content of CME activities. All relevant conflicts of interest that are identified are thoroughly vetted by EOCME for fair balance, scientific objectivity, and patient care recommendations. EOCME is committed to providing its learners with CME activities that promote improvements or quality in healthcare and not a specific proprietary business or a commercial interest.

**The planning committee, staff, authors and editors listed below have identified no financial relationships or relationships to products or devices they or their spouse/life partner have with commercial interest related to the content of this CME activity:**

Mahmoud I. Awad, MD; Regan W. Bergmark, MD; Nadim Bikhazi, MD; Daniel R. Cox, MD; Stacey T. Gray, MD; Natalia Hajnas, BA; Kristen Helm; Katherine Hicks, MD, MS; David W. Hsu, MD; Ashutosh Kacker, MD; Alison Kemp; Jessica McCool; Sam P. Most, MD; Christopher R. Roxbury, MD; Sheena Samra, MD; Theodore A. Schuman, MD; Janki Shah, MD; Raj Sindwani, MD, FACS; Matthew M. Smith, MD; Emily Spataro, MD; Jeffrey T. Steitz, MD; Jeffrey D. Suh, MD; Subhalakshmi Vaidyanathan; Jennifer A. Villwock, MD; Carol H. Yan, MD.

**The planning committee, staff, authors and editors listed below have identified financial relationships or relationships to products or devices they or their spouse/life partner have with commercial interest related to the content of this CME activity:**

**James H. Atkins:** is a consultant/advisor for Arrinex, Inc. and Acclarent, Inc.
**Peter H. Hwang, MD:** is a consultant/advisor for Arrinex, Inc.
**Stacey L. Ishman, MD, MPH:** is a consultant/advisor for Medtronic
**Ronald B. Kuppersmith, MD:** is a consultant/advisor for Entellus Medical, Inc. and Arrinex, Inc.
**Brent A. Senior, MD:** is a consultant/advisor for Spirox, Inc.
**Douglas Sidle, MD:** is a consultant/advisor for Spirox, Inc.
**Dean M. Toriumi, MD:** is a consultant/advisor Spirox, Inc.
**Sarah K. Wise, MD, MSCR:** is a consultant/advisor for Elron Electronics Industries Ltd., Medtronic, and OptiNose US, Inc.

## UNAPPROVED/OFF-LABEL USE DISCLOSURE

The EOCME requires CME faculty to disclose to the participants:
1. When products or procedures being discussed are off-label, unlabelled, experimental, and/or investigational (not US Food and Drug Administration [FDA] approved); and
2. Any limitations on the information presented, such as data that are preliminary or that represent ongoing research, interim analyses, and/or unsupported opinions. Faculty may discuss information about pharmaceutical agents that is outside of FDA-approved labelling. This information is intended solely for CME and is not intended to promote off-label use of these medications. If you have any questions, contact the medical affairs department of the manufacturer for the most recent prescribing information.

**TO ENROLL**

To enroll in the *Otolaryngologic Clinics of North America* Continuing Medical Education program, call customer service at 1-800-654-2452 or sign up online at http://www.theclinics.com/home/cme. The CME program is available to subscribers for an additional annual fee of USD 260.

**METHOD OF PARTICIPATION**

In order to claim credit, participants must complete the following:

1. Complete enrolment as indicated above.
2. Read the activity.
3. Complete the CME Test and Evaluation. Participants must achieve a score of 70% on the test. All CME Tests and Evaluations must be completed online.

**CME INQUIRIES/SPECIAL NEEDS**

For all CME inquiries or special needs, please contact elsevierCME@elsevier.com.

# Contributors

## CONSULTING EDITOR

**SUJANA S. CHANDRASEKHAR, MD, FACS, FAAOHNS**
Past President, American Academy of Otolaryngology–Head and Neck Surgery, Partner,
ENT & Allergy Associates, LLP, Clinical Professor, Department of Otolaryngology–Head
and Neck Surgery, Zucker School of Medicine at Hofstra-Northwell, Hempstead,
New York; Clinical Associate Professor, Department of Otolaryngology–Head and Neck
Surgery, Icahn School of Medicine at Mount Sinai, New York, New York, USA

## EDITORS

**JENNIFER A. VILLWOCK, MD**
Assistant Professor, Department of Otolaryngology–Head and Neck Surgery, University
of Kansas Medical Center, Kansas University, Kansas City, Kansas

**RONALD B. KUPPERSMITH, MD**
Professor, Department of Surgery, Texas A&M University Health Science Center, College
Station, Texas

## AUTHORS

**JAMES H. ATKINS, MD**
Texas Sinus Center, San Antonio, Texas

**MAHMOUD I. AWAD, MD**
Department of Otolaryngology–Head and Neck Surgery, Weill Cornell Medical College,
New York, New York

**REGAN W. BERGMARK, MD**
Gliklich Healthcare Innovation Scholar, Department of Otolaryngology–Head and Neck
Surgery, Massachusetts Eye and Ear, Department of Otolaryngology, Harvard Medical
School, Boston, Massachusetts

**NADIM BIKHAZI, MD**
Ogden Clinic, Ogden, Utah

**DANIEL R. COX, MD**
Rhinology Fellow, Clinical Instructor, Department of Otolaryngology–Head and Neck
Surgery, Emory University, Atlanta, Georgia

**STACEY T. GRAY, MD**
Associate Professor, Department of Otolaryngology–Head and Neck Surgery, Massachusetts
Eye and Ear, Department of Otolaryngology, Harvard Medical School, Boston, Massachusetts

**NATALIA HAJNAS, BA**
Medical Student, College of Medicine, University of Illinois at Chicago, Chicago, Illinois

**KATHERINE HICKS, MD, MS**
Resident Physician in Otolaryngology–Head and Neck Surgery, McGaw Medical Center of Northwestern University, Chicago, Illinois

**DAVID W. HSU, MD**
Rhinology Fellow, Clinical Instructor, UCLA Department of Head and Neck Surgery, Los Angeles, California

**PETER H. HWANG, MD**
Professor, Vice Chair of Clinical Affairs, Department of Otolaryngology–Head and Neck Surgery, Stanford University School of Medicine, Stanford, California

**STACEY L. ISHMAN, MD, MPH**
Director of Otolaryngology Outcomes Research, Professor, Departments of Otolaryngology and Pulmonary Medicine, Surgical Director, Upper Airway Center, Cincinnati Children's Hospital Medical Center, University of Cincinnati, Cincinnati, Ohio

**ASHUTOSH KACKER, MD, FACS**
Department of Otolaryngology–Head and Neck Surgery, Weill Cornell Medical College, New York, New York

**RONALD B. KUPPERSMITH, MD**
Professor, Department of Surgery, Texas A&M University Health Science Center, College Station, Texas

**SAM P. MOST, MD**
Division of Facial Plastic and Reconstructive Surgery, Stanford University School of Medicine, Stanford, California

**CHRISTOPHER R. ROXBURY, MD**
Head and Neck Institute, Cleveland Clinic, Cleveland, Ohio

**SHEENA SAMRA, MD**
Resident Physician, Department of Otolaryngology–Head and Neck Surgery, University of Illinois at Chicago, Chicago, Illinois

**THEODORE A. SCHUMAN, MD**
Assistant Professor, Rhinology, Allergy, and Skull Base Surgery, Department of Otolaryngology–Head and Neck Surgery, Virginia Commonwealth University, Richmond, Virginia

**BRENT A. SENIOR, MD**
Vice Chairman for Clinical Affairs, Nathaniel and Sheila Harris Distinguished Professor, Chief, Division of Rhinology, Allergy, and Skull Base Surgery, Professor of Otolaryngology and Neurosurgery, Department of Otolaryngology–Head and Neck Surgery, University of North Carolina at Chapel Hill, Chapel Hill, North Carolina

**JANKI SHAH, MD**
Resident Physician, Head and Neck Institute, Cleveland Clinic, Cleveland, Ohio

**DOUGLAS SIDLE, MD**
Assistant Professor of Otolaryngology–Head and Neck Surgery, McGaw Medical Center of Northwestern University, Chicago, Illinois

**RAJ SINDWANI, MD, FACS**
Vice Chairman, Section Head, Rhinology, Sinus, and Skull Base Surgery, Head & Neck Institute, Cleveland Clinic, Cleveland, Ohio

**MATTHEW M. SMITH, MD**
Clinical Fellow, Department of Pediatric Otolaryngology, Cincinnati Children's Hospital Medical Center, Cincinnati, Ohio

**EMILY SPATARO, MD**
Division of Facial Plastic and Reconstructive Surgery, Stanford University School of Medicine, Stanford, California

**JEFFREY T. STEITZ, MD**
AAFPRS Fellow, Division of Facial Plastic and Reconstructive Surgery, Department of Otolaryngology–Head and Neck Surgery, University of Illinois at Chicago, Chicago, Illinois

**JEFFREY D. SUH, MD**
Associate Professor, UCLA Department of Head and Neck Surgery, Los Angeles, California

**DEAN M. TORIUMI, MD**
Associate Professor, Department of Otolaryngology–Head and Neck Surgery, University of Illinois at Chicago, Chicago, Illinois

**JENNIFER A. VILLWOCK, MD**
Assistant Professor, Department of Otolaryngology–Head and Neck Surgery, University of Kansas Medical Center, Kansas University, Kansas City, Kansas

**SARAH K. WISE, MD, MSCR**
Associate Professor, Department of Otolaryngology–Head and Neck Surgery, Emory University, Atlanta, Georgia

**CAROL H. YAN, MD**
Clinical Instructor, Department of Otolaryngology–Head and Neck Surgery, Stanford University School of Medicine, Stanford, California

# Contents

**Erratum** xv

**Foreword: Appreciating the Intricacies of a Stuffy Nose** xvii

Sujana S. Chandrasekhar

**Preface: Nasal Airway Obstruction** xix

Jennifer A. Villwock and Ronald B. Kuppersmith

**Anatomy and Physiology of Nasal Obstruction** 853

David W. Hsu and Jeffrey D. Suh

Nasal obstruction is a common presenting symptom to clinicians and affects up to one-third of the population. There are several factors that cause nasal obstruction, including anatomic, physiologic, and pathophysiologic factors. The anatomy and physiology of nasal obstruction is complicated and is influenced by patency of nasal passages, mucociliary function, airflow receptors, autonomic function, and degree of mucosal inflammation. Common anatomic causes include internal nasal valve stenosis/collapse, septal deviation, and turbinate hypertrophy. Common physiologic causes include sinonasal inflammatory disorders and iatrogenic causes.

**Diagnostic Algorithm for Evaluating Nasal Airway Obstruction** 867

Jennifer A. Villwock and Ronald B. Kuppersmith

Nasal obstruction is a common symptom and can have a large impact on patient quality of life. There are numerous causes, including anatomic, congenital, inflammatory, infectious, neoplastic, toxic, and systemic. An algorithmic approach can aid in ensuring all pertinent patient information is incorporated into the final diagnosis and treatment plan. Key components include a thorough history, physical examination including modified Cottle and Cottle maneuver, patient-reported outcome measures and/or quality of life questionnaires, examination with and without decongestion, and nasal endoscopy. The resultant information can then be effectively used to narrow the differential and guide the next steps in management.

**Treatment Paradigm for Nasal Airway Obstruction** 873

Theodore A. Schuman and Brent A. Senior

Nasal airway obstruction (NAO) is a common otolaryngic complaint with many potential causes, frequently structural or inflammatory in nature. Patients typically have multiple coexisting factors leading to symptoms. Good patient outcomes require careful preoperative evaluation, including nasal endoscopy, to accurately identify sources of obstruction and tailor intervention appropriately. Common structural causes of NAO include inferior turbinate hypertrophy, nasal septal deviation, and narrowing or collapse of the internal or external nasal valves. The internal nasal valve has the narrowest cross-sectional area within the nasal airway and is thus most sensitive to changes in dimension due to anatomic variation or surgical intervention.

### Measuring Nasal Obstruction Outcomes

883

Emily Spataro and Sam P. Most

Methods of measuring nasal obstruction outcomes include both objective anatomic and physiologic measurements, as well as subjective patient-reported measures. Anatomic measurements include acoustic rhinometry, imaging studies, and clinician-derived examination findings. Physiologic measures include rhinomanometry, nasal peak inspiratory flow, and computational fluid dynamics. Patient-reported outcome measures (PROMs) are self-reported assessments of disease-specific quality-of-life outcomes. Several studies attempted correlation of these outcome measures; however, few show strong correlation. Expert opinion favors determining successful surgical outcomes using PROMs. This article provides a summary of current nasal obstruction outcome measures.

### Medical Treatment of Nasal Airway Obstruction

897

Daniel R. Cox and Sarah K. Wise

Nasal obstruction is a common, and potentially debilitating, problem. It is caused by a combination of structural factors and/or mucosal swelling/inflammation. The medical treatment of nasal obstruction is aimed at decreasing mucosal inflammation and edema and is generally guided by the underlying cause. Several different drug classes are commonly used in the treatment of nasal obstruction, each with different indications and pros and cons to their use. This article discusses the most commonly used therapies for nasal obstruction. Current evidence on the efficacy and side-effect profile of each therapy is reviewed.

### Techniques in Septoplasty: Traditional Versus Endoscopic Approaches

909

Janki Shah, Christopher R. Roxbury, and Raj Sindwani

This article provides a review of modern techniques in the surgical management of the deviated septum, with emphasis on the comparison of traditional versus endoscopic septoplasty approaches. Relevant anatomy and physiology of the nasal septum are discussed. A brief history of the evolution of the surgical approaches for the correction of a deviated septum is provided. Traditional and endoscopic septoplasty techniques are reviewed; the indications, advantages, and limitations of each approach are highlighted. Potential complications of septoplasty, with a focus on prevention and management, are also discussed.

### Surgical Management of Turbinate Hypertrophy

919

Regan W. Bergmark and Stacey T. Gray

Inferior turbinate reduction is a common technique used to improve nasal breathing in patients with inferior turbinate hypertrophy. Subjective nasal breathing improves for the majority of patients with most surgical techniques, but effectiveness often diminishes over time. Inferior turbinate reduction techniques typically have low complication rates. Empty nose syndrome is a rare complication associated most classically with total or subtotal inferior turbinate reduction. Most techniques attempt to preserve the turbinate mucosa for the purposes of preserving normal mucociliary clearance and sensation. Clinical trials comparing inferior turbinate reduction techniques as well as studies on long-term effectiveness, value, and cost are needed.

### Surgical Management of Nasal Valve Collapse        929

Sheena Samra, Jeffrey T. Steitz, Natalia Hajnas, and Dean M. Toriumi

Nasal valve collapse has multiple causes, including congenital, traumatic, and, unfortunately, iatrogenic. Recognition of the causes of nasal valve collapse and the methodology for treatment is paramount not only for the otolaryngologist but also for any physician managing the nasal airway. This article focuses on the cause and surgical management of internal and external nasal valve collapse.

### Surgical Management of Nonallergic Rhinitis        945

Carol H. Yan and Peter H. Hwang

Nonallergic rhinitis (NAR) describes chronic symptoms of nasal congestion, obstruction, and rhinorrhea unrelated to a specific allergen based on skin or serum testing. Vasomotor rhinitis is the most frequent subtype of NAR. Although medical management is the first-line treatment of NAR, there is a role for surgical therapy when medications fail to improve symptoms. Surgical options for NAR include inferior turbinate reduction and botulinum toxin injection as well as more directed targeting of the autonomic nerve supply to the nasal cavity through vidian neurectomy, posterior nasal neurectomy, and cryoablation of the posterior nerve.

### Office-Based Procedures for Nasal Airway Obstruction        957

Nadim Bikhazi and James H. Atkins

Treatment of common rhinologic problems with in-office surgical procedures has increased dramatically in response to patient preference, evolving insurance patterns, and changes in coding and reimbursement. Because this is an emerging practice, there is not a lot of evidence published about how to best perform these techniques. This article provides practical advice from experienced surgeons related to logistics and anesthetic techniques for conducting in-office surgical treatment of nasal airway obstruction, an overview of office setup and necessary equipment, and specific procedural considerations. Attention is also paid to pharmacologic issues. Logistics and clinical considerations for common office-based procedures for obstructive pathology are reviewed.

### Pediatric Nasal Obstruction        971

Matthew M. Smith and Stacey L. Ishman

Nasal obstruction is one of the most common problems seen by pediatric otolaryngologists. Prompt treatment of nasal obstruction can be critical in newborns and infants because of their obligatory nasal breathing.

Older children will typically have more inflammatory, infectious, or traumatic causes of nasal obstruction. Nasal obstruction can lead to a significant decrease in the quality of life in children along with an increase in health care expenditures.

**Nasal Obstruction Considerations in Cosmetic Rhinoplasty**                    987

Douglas Sidle and Katherine Hicks

Cosmetic rhinoplasty is an increasingly popular procedure in the United States. There are critical aspects of preoperative planning and intraoperative execution that facilitate successful rhinoplasty. Thorough preoperative assessment of the structures comprising the internal and external nasal valves and identification of potential at-risk areas for static or dynamic compromise must be done before surgery. Thoughtful maneuvers and meticulous surgical technique must be used. Postoperative counseling ranges from simple reassurance to medical therapy to procedural efforts to alleviate a patient's concerns. It is important to establish rapport with the patient and dutifully address all cosmetic and functional concerns.

**Nasal Obstruction Considerations in Sleep Apnea**                    1003

Mahmoud I. Awad and Ashutosh Kacker

Obstructive sleep apnea (OSA) is a highly prevalent condition in the context of the global obesity epidemic with significant medical comorbidities and psychosocial implications. The first-line treatment of OSA is continuous positive airway pressure (CPAP). There is evidence to demonstrate an association between nasal obstruction and OSA. Therefore, medications and surgical interventions to address nasal obstruction may play a role in the treatment of OSA. In addition, surgical correction of nasal obstruction has been shown to improve CPAP tolerance and compliance.

# OTOLARYNGOLOGIC CLINICS OF NORTH AMERICA

**FORTHCOMING ISSUES**

*December 2018*
**Facial Palsy: Diagnostic and Therapeutic Management**
Teresa M. O, Nate Jowett, and
Tessa Hadlock, *Editors*

*February 2019*
**Patient Safety**
Rahul Shah, *Editor*

*April 2019*
**Implantable Auditory Devices**
Darius Kohan and
Sujana S. Chandrasekhar, *Editors*

**RECENT ISSUES**

*August 2018*
**Geriatric Otolaryngology**
Natasha Mirza and Jennifer Y. Lee, *Editors*

*June 2018*
**Global Health in Otolaryngology**
James E. Saunders, Susan R. Cordes,
and Mark E. Zafereo, *Editors*

*April 2018*
**Otosclerosis and Stapes Surgery**
Adrien A. Eshraghi and Fred F. Telischi,
*Editors*

**SERIES OF RELATED INTEREST**

*Facial Plastic Surgery Clinics*
www.facialplastic.theclinics.com
*Surgical Clinics*
www.surgical.theclinics.com

**THE CLINICS ARE AVAILABLE ONLINE!**
Access your subscription at:
www.theclinics.com

# Erratum

An error was made in the June 2018 issue of *Otolaryngologic Clinics* (Volume 51, Issue 3) in the article, "Regional Overview of Specific Populations, Workforce Considerations, Training and Diseases in Latin America" by Drs. J. Pablo Stolovitzky and Jacqueline Alvarado.

Table 2 on page 655 states that the population in Chile is 8,357,784 with 500 ORL and 6.0 ORL per 100,000 inhabitants. It should state that the population in Chile is 18,357,784 with 500 ORL and 2.7 ORL per 100,000 inhabitants.

The online version of the article has been corrected.

Otolaryngol Clin N Am 51 (2018) xv
https://doi.org/10.1016/j.otc.2018.07.016
0030-6665/18/© 2018 Elsevier Inc. All rights reserved.

oto.theclinics.com

# Foreword

# Appreciating the Intricacies of a Stuffy Nose

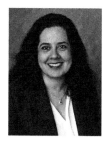

Sujana S. Chandrasekhar, MD, FACS, FAAOHNS
*Consulting Editor*

Common conditions occur commonly, but identifying the causes and optimizing treatment may be difficult. Nasal airway obstruction, one of the most common complaints related to Otolaryngology, is often reported to health care providers in various fields. These include pediatrics, family practice, internal medicine, geriatrics, obstetrics/gynecology, emergency medicine, and, of course, otolaryngology. Anyone who's spent a sleepless night due to a blocked nose or had difficulty speaking during the day or managing the secondary dry mouth/throat that comes with a significantly obstructed nasal cavity can appreciate the dramatic reduction in quality of life that results from this chronic condition.

Drs Villwock and Kuppersmith, the Guest Editors of this issue of *Otolaryngologic Clinics of North America*, have compiled a thorough series of articles written by experts/key opinion leaders that explore this problem from anatomy and physiology through evaluation and to treatment of "simple" cases to ones complicated by comorbidities. Each article flows from the previous one and also stands alone.

Anatomical dissections of the nose and nasopharynx make up some of the earliest knowledge we have. Drs Hsu and Suh relate that established data to modern appreciation of the structure and the function of the nose. Understanding this allows us to see where things might go wrong. Drs Villwock and Kuppersmith have an excellent algorithm to follow, to enable accurate diagnosis, avoid incorrect or missed diagnoses, and streamline that process. Immediately follows a similarly logical treatment paradigm by Drs Schuman and Senior. Again, the patient is best benefited by receiving appropriate and targeted care and avoiding incorrect interventions.

"Doctor, my nose is stuffy" is a difficult statement to quantify. Drs Spataro and Most detail how outcomes can be measured and incorporated into the medical chart, so as to be able to improve performance and outcomes for both the individual physician and patient, and as we review larger sets of these data. Knowing the gamut of appropriate

Otolaryngol Clin N Am 51 (2018) xvii–xviii
https://doi.org/10.1016/j.otc.2018.06.003
0030-6665/18/© 2018 Published by Elsevier Inc.

medical interventions, their side-effect profiles, and the likelihood of success, as well as how long to attempt these noninvasive techniques, is important and is detailed nicely by Drs Cox and Wise.

One of the most attractive aspects of Otolaryngology, to me, is the ability to be both the medical and surgical physician for any given problem. If the patient does not experience adequate relief from appropriate medical treatment, or if there is an obvious structural issue from the onset, the articles in this issue detailing the various surgical options discuss what can and should be done, given the findings. These procedures include septoplasty, reduction of turbinate hypertrophy, management of nasal valve collapse, and surgery of nonallergic rhinitis. In addition, there are office-based procedures that can be done with minimal discomfort and time lost to the patient. I urge you to read these five articles as they provide succinct but thorough explanations of these treatments.

Special populations include children, individuals undergoing cosmetic rhinoplasty, and patients with obstructive sleep apnea. The articles addressing these are also "must-reads," in order to avoid missing opportunities for dramatic improvements in rhinologic quality of life for these individuals.

Again, I commend Drs Villwock and Kuppersmith and all of the authors on this robust issue of *Otolaryngologic Clinics of North America* on Nasal Airway Obstruction. I hope that you enjoy it and find it to be helpful in your practice.

Sujana S. Chandrasekhar, MD, FACS, FAAOHNS
ENT & Allergy Associates, LLP
18 East 48th Street, 2nd Floor
New York, NY 10017, USA

Zucker School of Medicine at Hofstra-Northwell
Hempstead, NY 11549, USA

Icahn School of Medicine at Mount Sinai
New York, NY 10029, USA

*E-mail address:*
ssc@nyotology.com

# Preface

# Nasal Airway Obstruction

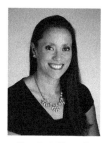
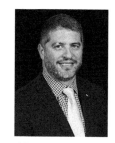

Jennifer A. Villwock, MD    Ronald B. Kuppersmith, MD
*Editors*

Nasal airway obstruction has a significant impact on quality of life and is one of the most common complaints of patients seeking treatment from Otolaryngologist–Head and Neck Surgeons. While nasal airway obstruction is common, its causes can be multifactorial. Focused treatment can help alleviate obstruction while minimizing unnecessary interventions. This issue of *Otolaryngologic Clinics of North America* is designed to provide a comprehensive overview of the diagnosis, medical and surgical management options, and methods of measuring the extent of initial obstruction and response to nasal airway obstruction treatment.

Drs Hsu and Suh review the anatomy and physiology relevant to nasal obstruction, which informs the underlying causes and areas of consideration that may be important during intervention. We, Drs Villwock and Kuppersmith, detail critical elements to consider while evaluating patients with nasal airway obstruction. Drs Schuman and Senior provide a treatment paradigm for approaching patients with nasal airway obstruction. One of the biggest challenges related to nasal airway obstruction is measurement of its severity. While the symptoms are subjective, objective measures have been elusive, making the diagnosis and measurement of outcomes difficult to standardize. Drs Spataro and Most summarize methods that have been tried and methods that are currently available.

With respect to treatment, Drs Cox and Wise summarize currently available medical treatments. The effective use of medications requires a thorough evaluation and effort to educate patients about the purpose, benefits, and risks of available pharmaceuticals. Surgical interventions for nasal obstruction typically involve procedures aimed at the septum, turbinates, and/or nasal valve. Drs Shah, Roxbury, and Sindwani describe both traditional and endoscopic septoplasty. Drs Bergmark and Gray provide an overview of the evidence for turbinate surgery and the different methods that can be utilized. Drs Samra, Steitz, and Toriumi address the primary surgical management of nasal valve collapse. While most physicians are focused on anatomic and

Otolaryngol Clin N Am 51 (2018) xix–xx
https://doi.org/10.1016/j.otc.2018.06.002
0030-6665/18/© 2018 Published by Elsevier Inc.

oto.theclinics.com

inflammatory causes of nasal obstruction, Drs Yan and Hwang provide an update on neurogenic causes of nasal symptoms, which may easily be overlooked, and surgical approaches for managing this challenging problem. Drs Bihkazi and Atkins share important insight for physicians wishing to perform their interventions in an office setting rather than under general anesthesia in an operative suite.

There are several special instances in which the management of nasal obstruction needs to be considered. Drs Smith and Ishman examine issues specific to the diagnosis and management of pediatric nasal airway obstruction. Drs Sidle and Hicks discuss how cosmetic rhinoplasty can affect nasal obstruction and approaches to minimize nasal obstruction as an outcome of these procedures. Dr Awad and Kacker address the role of nasal obstruction in patients with poor sleep quality and sleep apnea, common and challenging problems.

We believe this issue provides a summary of the current state-of-the-art treatment of nasal airway obstruction. We would like to express our gratitude to the contributing authors for their efforts.

Jennifer A. Villwock, MD
Department of Otolaryngology
Head and Neck Surgery
Kansas University
University of Kansas Medical Center
3901 Rainbow Boulevard, MS 3010
Kansas City, KS 66160, USA

Ronald B. Kuppersmith, MD
Department of Surgery
Texas A&M Health Science Center
1730 Birmingham Drive
College Station, TX 77845, USA

*E-mail addresses:*
jvillwock@kumc.edu (J.A. Villwock)
rbk@texasentandallergy.com (R.B. Kuppersmith)

# Anatomy and Physiology of Nasal Obstruction

David W. Hsu, MD, Jeffrey D. Suh, MD*

## KEYWORDS

- Nasal obstruction • Deviated septum • Nasal valve collapse • Turbinate hypertrophy
- Nasal cycle

## KEY POINTS

- The cause of nasal obstruction is caused by a wide array of anatomic, physiologic, pathophysiologic, and iatrogenic factors; it can often be multifactorial.
- Optimal nasal airflow is determined by patent nasal passages, intact mucociliary function, normal functioning receptors for airflow, and degree of mucosal inflammation.
- The internal nasal valve comprises the area of greatest overall resistance to airflow and is affected by Bernoulli forces and Poiseuille law.
- The septum and turbinates are common anatomic causes for nasal obstruction but are easily treatable.
- Nasal obstruction in rhinitis and sinusitis are caused by aberrant inflammatory responses.

## INTRODUCTION

Nasal obstruction is a common presenting symptom to both primary care physicians and otolaryngologists and may be caused by a wide range of anatomic, physiologic, and pathophysiologic factors. Up to one-third of the population complains of nasal obstruction and seeks treatment from their physicians.[1] In this article, the authors discuss the anatomy and physiology of nasal obstruction.

The human nose is evolutionarily adapted to warm, humidify, and filter inspired air before its reaching the pulmonary system. In this way, the nose and lungs work together as a unified airway. The nose also plays an important role in combating inhaled foreign particles and detecting odorants for olfaction. It has evolved to bring in a large volume of air through the nostrils and nasal cavities while also maximizing the air's contact with mucosal areas.[2] These adaptations include increased nasal projection, anterior nasal convexity, exaggerated nasal angles, anterior nasal spine prominence, and an intricate nasal cartilaginous tip.[3]

Disclosure Statement: The authors have nothing to disclose.
UCLA Department of Head and Neck Surgery, 200 UCLA Medical Plaza, Suite 550, Los Angeles, CA 90095, USA
* Corresponding author.
E-mail address: jeffsuh@mednet.ucla.edu

Otolaryngol Clin N Am 51 (2018) 853–865
https://doi.org/10.1016/j.otc.2018.05.001
0030-6665/18/© 2018 Elsevier Inc. All rights reserved.

oto.theclinics.com

Optimal nasal airflow requires (1) patent nasal passages, (2) intact mucociliary function, (3) normal functioning receptors for airflow, and (4) absence of mucosal inflammation. Any aberration of these factors can lead to the sensation of decreased airflow. Air contacts the nasal mucous membranes as it flows through the nasal valve, travels past the septum and turbinates, and finally flows through the nasopharynx. Anatomic changes can disrupt this flow, thus causing resistance and subsequent nasal obstruction.

As the air flows through the nose, the turbinates induce nonlaminar flow and air temperature changes that are sensed by trigeminal cool thermoreceptors, which then regulate the sensation of airflow and nasal patency.[4] Other receptors such as pain receptors or mechanoreceptors may also play a role. Any dysfunction of the mucociliary function or airflow receptors will adversely affect nasal airflow and cause the sensation of decreased air passage.

Anatomic causes of nasal obstruction include internal or external nasal valve stenosis/collapse, septal deviations, an enlarged septal swell body, inferior turbinate hypertrophy, choanal stenosis/atresia, nasopharyngeal obstruction, and iatrogenic scarring. Physiologic causes include the natural nasal cycle, changes in the nasal autonomic nervous system, and sinonasal inflammatory conditions.

## NASAL ANATOMY
### Skin/Soft Tissue Envelope

Overlying the skeletal framework of the nose is the skin-soft tissue envelope (SSTE).[5] The skin of the nose varies in thickness going from superior to inferior along the nose. The skin is thickest at the nasion, which denotes the bony junction of the frontal bone with the 2 nasal bones. The SSTE is thinnest at the rhinion, which is the osseocartilaginous junction of the caudal edge of the nasal bones and cephalic edge of the upper lateral cartilage (ULC). The skin does thicken along the dorsum as it descends from the rhinion to the nasal tip, where sebaceous glands reside.

The subcutanenous layer of the nose is composed of a superficial fatty layer, a fibromuscular layer, a deep fatty layer, and periosteum and/or perichrondrium.[5] Importantly, the fibromuscular layer is the nasal subcutaneous muscular aponeurosis system (SMAS), which connects with the SMAS layer of the face and encases the mimetic muscles of the nose.[5]

Deep to the SSTE is the investing nasal musculature. Elevator muscles include the procerus, levator labii superioris alaeque nasi, and anomalous nasi. Depressor muscles are the alar nasalis and depressor septi nasi. Compressor muscles include the transverse nasalis and compressor narium minor. And finally, dilator naris anterior is a minor dilator muscle.

The internal nasal lining consists of keratinizing squamous cell epithelium at the nasal vestibule. Once inside the nasal cavity, the surfaces are composed of pseudostratified ciliated columnar respiratory cells. Seromucinous glands are also abundantly found in the sinonasal cavity.

### Nasal Bony Framework

The framework of the nose is commonly divided into thirds: the upper third comprises the osseous nasal vault made up by the nasal bones, the middle third defined by the ULCs, and the lower third defined by the lower lateral cartilages (LLCs) (**Fig. 1**A).[6]

The osseous vault forms a pyramidal structure and consists of the paired nasal bones attaching superiorly to the frontal bone and laterally to the frontal process of the maxilla.[5] This bone framework along with the bony septum provides the principal

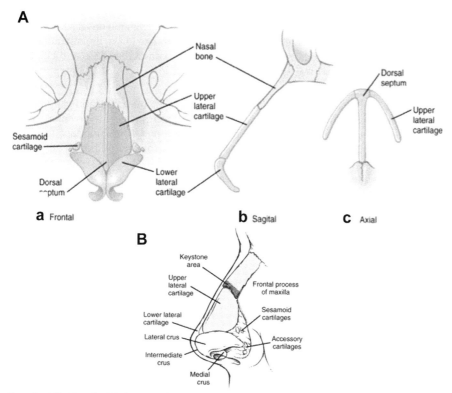

**Fig. 1.** (*A*) Nasal thirds: nasal bones represent upper nasal third, upper lateral cartilages represent the middle third, and lower lateral cartilages represent the lower third. (a – frontal view, b – sagittal view, c – axial view). (*B*) Keystone area: the strong fibrous connection between the nasal bones and the upper lateral cartilages provides stability to the nose. (*From* [A] McCarn KE, Downs BW, Cook TA, et al. The middle vault: upper lateral cartilage modifications. In: Azizzadeh B, Murphy MR, Johnson CM, et al, editors. Master techniques in rhinoplasty. Philadelphia: Saunders; 2011. p. 159–67, with permission; and [B] Chegar BE, Tatum, SA. Nasal fractures. In: Flint PW, Haughey BH, Lund V, et al, editors. Cummings otolaryngology. Philadelphia: Saunders; 2015. p. 494, with permission.)

support of the nose. The caudal or free edge of the osseous vault forms the superior portion of the pyriform aperture, and more importantly, the keystone area of the nose is where it articulates with the nasal septum (**Fig. 1**B).

### Nasal Cartilage

The nasal cartilages make up the middle and lower thirds of the nose. The upper cartilaginous vault or middle third is composed of paired ULCs (see **Fig. 1**A). The UCLs are triangular, shieldlike structures that are fused midline to the dorsal edge of the cartilaginous septum.[6] Laterally, the ULCs approach the pyriform aperture and fuse with dense fibrous tissue. The caudal edge attaches to the LLC and this area is called the scroll. Most importantly, the caudal edge of the ULC, along with the nasal septum, floor of the nose, and head of the inferior turbinate, forms the internal nasal valve.[7]

The lower third of the nose or the lower cartilaginous vault is composed of the paired LLCs. The shape and configuration of these cartilages determine the nasal tip and nasal base. The LLCs are divided into 3 sections: the medial crus, the intermediate crus, and the lateral crus. Most importantly, the LLCs along with the nasal septum provide nasal tip support. Specifically, the major tip supports are LLCs, the attachment of the medial crura to the caudal septum, and the scroll area of the ULCs and LLCs.[5]

### Nasal Septum

The nasal septum functions to support the structure of the nose and may cause disruption of nasal airflow when significantly deformed. In fact, a deviated nasal septum is the most common cause of nasal obstruction.[1] It is important to recall that septal deformities are common, but not often symptomatic. Although some patients with a deviated septum and nasal obstruction may have a history of nasal trauma, the majority do not have a clear inciting event. Birth trauma or microfractures early in life have been implicated in causing aberrant growth of the septum.[8]

From anterior to posterior, the anatomy of the nasal septum is composed of[1] a membranous,[2] a cartilaginous, and[3] an osseous component (**Fig. 2**A). The membranous component is composed of fibrofatty tissue and located between the columella and the quadrangular cartilage. The septal cartilage is primarily composed of the quadrangular cartilage. The posterior nasal septum is composed of the perpendicular plate of ethmoid, the nasal crest of palatine and maxillary bones, and the vomer.

### Septal Swell Body

The nasal septal swell body (NSB) is a widened region of the anterior nasal septum that is located anterior to the middle turbinate (**Fig. 2**B). This region is referred to as the

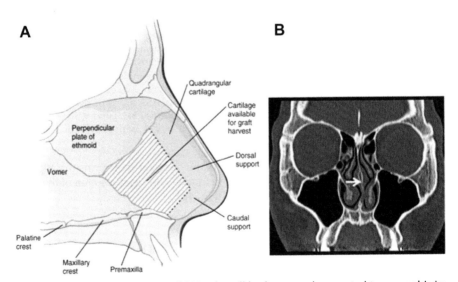

**Fig. 2.** (*A*) Nasal septum anatomy. (*B*) Nasal swell body: coronal computed tomographic image showing the nasal swell body (*arrow*). (*From* [*A*] Sarkissian RD. Cartilage grafting in rhinoplasty and nasal reconstruction. In: Azizzadeh B, Murphy MR, Johnson CM, et al, editors. Master techniques in rhinoplasty. Philadelphia: Saunders; 2011. p. 143–57, with permission; and [*B*] Koo SK, Kim JD, Moon JS, et al. The incidence of concha bullosa, unusual anatomic variation and its relationship to nasal septal deviation: a retrospective radiologic study. Auris Nasus Larynx 2017;44(5):561–70, with permission.)

septal turbinate and should not be confused with a septal deviation.[9] The NSB consists of cartilage and bone and is near the distal area of the internal nasal valve, which potentially provides a site of anatomic obstruction. Studies have shown that there is a high proportion of venous sinusoids similar to the inferior turbinate and both glandular and vasoerectile tissue in this area, which could all potentially alter nasal airflow.[10]

## Turbinates

The three-paired nasal turbinates, and their respective meati, are important landmarks of the lateral nasal wall. The superior and middle turbinates arise from the ethmoid bone, whereas the inferior turbinates are made of an independent bony structure. The turbinates are typically thin bone with adherent mucoperiosteum. However, the submucosal component of the inferior turbinate can hypertrophy in response to chronic allergen or irritant exposure. Similarly, the middle turbinate is also capable of undergoing polypoid degeneration.

The inferior turbinate helps regulate nasal airflow. It functions to maximize the intranasal surface area and facilitate humidification and warming of inspired air.[11] The inferior turbinate contains a rich supply in vascular channels that can engorge with blood depending on autonomic function.

Anatomic changes of the inferior turbinate help to explain its effect on nasal obstruction. Any changes in the cross-sectional area of the nasal valve, such as minor increases in inferior turbinate congestion, can significantly increase resistance. Also, histologic studies have shown that the medial aspect of the inferior turbinate is thicker and has more surface area than the lateral aspect.[12]

There are 3 anatomic variations (bony, soft tissue, and mixed) of the inferior turbinate that can narrow the nasal passage. Bony hypertrophy can be caused by a prominent inferolateral turn, and progressive ossification of the bone has also been described.[12] Soft tissue hypertrophy is very common and is usually seen in the setting of chronic inferior turbinate congestion as seen in chronic rhinitis (**Fig. 3**A). A mix of soft tissue and bony hypertrophy can also be seen in chronic rhinitis. Pneumatization of inferior turbinates is rare but can occur.

The middle turbinate serves as an important surgical landmark, but is a lesser causative agent for nasal resistance. A concha bullosa represents pneumatization of the middle turbinate. It is a common anatomic variant and found in approximately 25% of the population.[13] Conchae can be both bilateral and unilateral and most are usually small and asymptomatic (**Fig. 3**B). Unilateral cases are associated with septal deflections toward the contralateral side. If large enough, conchae bullosae can contribute to increased nasal airflow resistance.

Another anatomic variant of the middle turbinate is a paradoxic middle turbinate, which may cause nasal obstruction (**Fig. 3**C). This variant has an inferomedially curved free edge with a concave surface adjacent to the septum. When bulbous, a paradoxic middle turbinate can narrow the middle meatus, cause ostiomeatal complex blockage, and lead to nasal obstruction.

## Nasal Valve

The nasal valve is divided into an internal and external nasal valve; the internal nasal valve is the narrowest portion of the nasal airway.[14] This anatomic area comprises the area of greatest overall resistance to airflow.[15] The anatomic boundaries are composed of the dorsal nasal septum medially, the caudal edge of the ULC laterally, and anterior head of the inferior turbinate posteriorly (**Fig. 4**). The normal angle between the nasal septum and ULC is 10° to 15°.[16] Narrowing of this area is associated

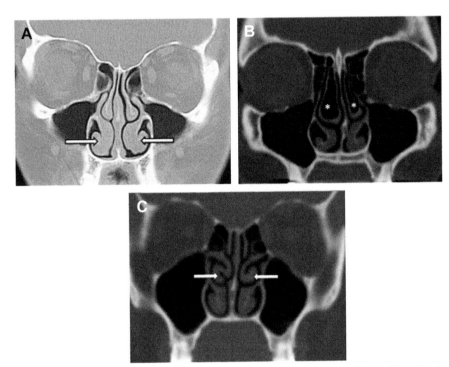

**Fig. 3.** (*A*) Coronal computed tomography (CT) with bilateral inferior turbinate hypertrophy (*arrows*), primarily soft tissue. (*B*) Coronal CT with bilateral concha bullosa (*asterisks*). (*C*) Coronal CT with bilateral paradoxic middle turbinate (*arrows*). (*From* Neskey D, Eloy JA, Casiano RR. Nasal, septal, and turbinate anatomy and embryology. Otolaryngol Clin North Am 2009;42(2):193–205; with permission.)

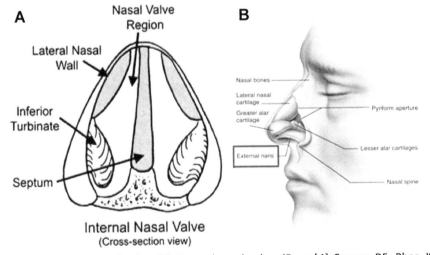

**Fig. 4.** (*A*) Internal nasal valve. (*B*) External nasal valve. (*From* [*A*] Cannon DE, Rhee JS. Evidence-based practice. Otolaryngol Clin North Am 2012;45(5):1033–43, with permission; and [*B*] Egan KK, Kim D, Kezirian EJ. Nasal obstruction and sleep-disordered breathing. In: Friedman M, editor. Sleep apnea and snoring. China: Elsevier; 2009. p. 120–3; with permission.)

with nasal obstruction because the internal nasal valve is responsible for approximately two-thirds of total nasal airway resistance.[14]

The external nasal valve, also known as the nasal vestibule under the nasal ala, is bounded by the medial crura of the alar cartilages, the alar rim, the nasal sill, and the membranous septum (see **Fig. 4**B). This is the first area in which airflow resistance may occur. Nasal airway obstruction at this level can be caused by severe nasal tip ptosis, deformation, redundancy, or weakness of the alar cartilages, or other anatomic anomalies.

## Choana

The choana, also known as the posterior nasal aperture, is the area that separates the nasal cavity from the nasopharynx and is delineated by the location of the posterior aspects of the septum and inferior turbinates. The choana is a space defined by the horizontal plate of the palatine bone anteriorly and inferiorly, the sphenoid bone superiorly and posteriorly, and the medial pterygoid plates laterally. In the midline, it is separated by the vomer. This area most commonly causes nasal obstruction in newborns with choanal atresia[17] but potentially can cause nasal obstruction in adults as well.

## Nasopharynx

The nasopharynx is the region where the nasal cavity and superior most part of pharynx meet. The area is delineated by the posterior nasal aperture anteriorly, mucosa overlying the superior pharyngeal constrictor muscles posteriorly, the mucoperiosteum of the upper clivus superiorly, and the soft palate inferiorly.[18]

The lateral boundaries of the nasopharynx are the Eustachian tube and the fossa of Rosenmuller, which lies between the Eustachian tube and posterior wall of the nasopharynx. Potential causes of nasal obstruction in this area include adenoid hypertrophy, scarring from previous surgery or neoplastic processes, such as nasopharyngeal carcinoma.

## Blood Supply

Terminal branches of the external and internal carotid arteries supply the extremely rich blood supply of the nasal cavity (**Fig. 5**A). The terminal branches of the external carotid artery system are the facial artery, which gives off the superior labial artery for the anterior nasal septum, and the internal maxillary artery, which courses within the pterygopalatine fossa to give the main blood supply to the nasal cavity.[19] The branches of the internal maxillary artery are the sphenopalatine, descending palatine, and infraorbital arteries. The sphenopalatine artery branches into conchal (posterolateral) and septal (posteromedial) branches. Lastly, the descending palatine artery becomes the greater palatine artery after it passes through the greater palatine canal and enters the nose through the incisive foramen. Once in the nose, the greater palatine artery supplies the anterior inferior septum.

The terminal branches of the internal carotid artery that give blood supply to the nasal cavity are the anterior and posterior ethmoid branches of the ophthalmic artery.[19] They both are found along the skull base and give blood supply to the septum. Where several branches of the external and internal carotid anastomose at the caudal end of the septum is an area called Kiesselbach or Little area (**Fig. 5**B).

## Sensory Innervation of Nose

The innervation of the nose is supplied by terminal branches of the first 2 divisions of the trigeminal nerve (cranial nerve V): the ophthalmic (V1) and maxillary (V2) nerves.

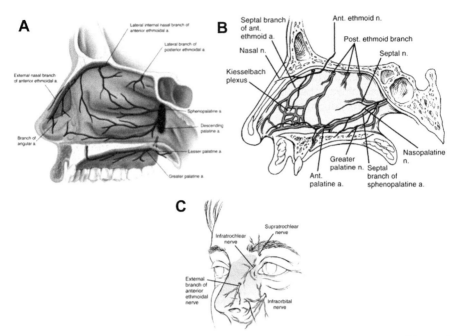

Fig. 5. (A) Arterial supply of nasal cavity. (B) Vasculature and sensory innervation of internal nasal cavity. Kiesselbach plexus represents the confluences of terminal branches of the external and internal carotid arteries in the nose. (C) Sensory innervation of external nose. (*From* [A] Baker SR. Reconstruction of the nose. In: Baker SR, editor. Local flaps in facial reconstruction. Philadelphia: Saunder; 2014. p. 415–80, with permission; and [B] Kridel R, Sturm-O'brien A. Nasal septum. In: Flint PW, Haughey BH, Lund V, et al, editors. Cummings otolaryngology. Philadelphia: Saunders; 2015. p. 474–92, with permission; and [C] Chegar BE, Tatum SA. Nasal fractures. In: Flint PW, Haughey BH, Lund V, et al, editors. Cummings otolaryngology. Philadelphia: Saunders; 2015. p. 493–505, with permission.)

These trigeminal fibers provide sensations of pain, temperature, and touch. The nasal intervention can be divided into the external nose and into the internal nose.

For the superior aspect of the external nose and the nasal tip, infratrochlear nerve (V1), the supratrochlear nerve (V1), and the external nasal branch of the anterior ethmoid nerve (V1) are responsible for innervation[20] (**Fig. 5**C). The inferior and lateral aspects of the nose are supplied by the infraorbital nerve (V2).

For the internal nasal cavity, the anterior and posterior ethmoid nerves (V1) innervate the superior lateral nasal wall. The sphenopalatine ganglion (V2) supplies the posterior nasal cavity and lateral nasal wall. The septum receives its supply from both the V1 and V2 branches of the internal nasal cavity.

In addition to the sensory innervation of the internal nasal cavity, there is an autonomic component to the nasal mucosa that will be discussed later in this article. Lastly, the special sensory branches of the cranial nerve I at the cribriform plate provide olfaction as well as parts of the superior turbinate and superior aspects of the septum.

### Characteristics of Nasal Mucosa

Nasal mucosa is composed of pseudostratified ciliated columnar respiratory cells, goblet cells, and the submucosal glands. This lining functions to create a moist, mucus-covered surface (mucous blanket) to trap harmful particles and mobilize them back toward the nasopharynx.[21]

The function of the nasal mucosa is to provide mucociliary transport (MCT) and ensure healthy airway surfaces.[21] A surface liquid overlies the nasal mucosa and is composed of 2 layers: the periciliary layer and the mucus layer. The *periciliary layer* provides an optimal environment for ciliary beating, whereas the *mucus layer* on top of it is the secretory product of the goblet cells and the submucosal glands.

Mucociliary clearance in the nasal cavity is driven by the coordinated beating of ciliated cells to clear inhaled foreign particles trapped in the mucus layers. The MCT helps clear out allergens and microbes. By this mechanism, mucus is transported from the respiratory tracts into the pharynx to prevent upper respiratory infections. Prolonged mucociliary clearance transit times are associated with sinus symptomatology and pathology. Dysfunction of MCT due to ciliary dysfunction can be seen in primary ciliary dyskinesia, increased viscosity of secretions as in cystic fibrosis or in inflammation seen in infections or allergies. This ultimately can lead to nasal obstruction and/or sinusitis.

## PHYSIOLOGY
### Nasal Airflow/Resistance

During inspiration, the air passes through the vestibule of the nose, flows through the narrow valve, disperses in the nasal cavity, and finally funnels through the nasopharynx. The structures within the nasal cavity cause nonlaminar flow, thus decelerating airflow and beneficially allowing air conditioning of inspired air. However, after a certain point, which varies by individual, such disruptions cease to be beneficial and cause nasal obstruction.

Patency of the nasal cavity relies on several components to counteract the potential of air resistance. Bernoulli forces favor the collapse of the nasal valve because high-velocity airflow can cause a decrease in intraluminal pressure and a subsequent vacuum effect.[14] Thus, the resiliency of the ULC and LLC is important to prevent collapse in this area. The inherent structure of the cartilage can be weakened with aging or previous surgery.

Poiseuille law best explains the effect of a decrease in nasal diameter on airflow. This law states that airflow is proportional to the radius of the airway raised to the fourth power.[14] As such, an anatomic narrowing caused by any of the 3 components of the internal nasal valve can have a dramatic effect on airflow. For example, trauma, such as in a previous rhinoplasty, especially in cases of overly aggressive lateral osteotomies, is a common cause. However, some patients may present with a narrowed nasal vault without a major anatomic abnormality.

### Nasal Cycle

The nasal cycle is a phenomenon of cyclic unilateral nasal cavity congestion due to an asymmetry of blood flow and engorgement of erectile tissue in the anterior part of the nasal septum and inferior turbinate.[22] The nasal cycle periodicity ranges from 25 minute to 8 hours. During waking hours, the average interval is between 1.5 and 4 hours.[22] In sensitive patients, this periodic congestion can cause fluctuating sensations of asymmetric nasal obstruction throughout the day. The nasal cycle is affected by physical exertion, changes with age, or positional changes.

The physiologic mechanisms that drive the nasal cycle are not well understood but are related to fluctuations in the autonomic nervous systems. Unilateral sympathetic dominance will facilitate vasoconstriction and decongestion in one nostril, whereas simultaneous parasympathetic function will cause vasodilation and congestion on the contralateral side.[22] Asymmetry of brain function and physiologic changes in heart rate, blood pressure, and blood glucose levels have also been implicated in regulating the nasal cycle.[22]

### Autonomic Innervation of Nasal Cavity

The autonomic nervous system controls the degree of vascular tone, level of congestion, and production of secretions in the nasal cavity.[23] Imbalance between the parasympathetic and sympathetic nervous system that favors the parasympathetic may result in increased turbinate congestion and symptomatic nasal obstruction. Furthermore, the parasympathetic nervous system regulates the air conditioning action, nasal resistance, and mucociliary function of the turbinates.

Presynaptic parasympathetic fibers travel along the greater superficial petrosal nerve after passing through the geniculate ganglion. They join the deep petrosal nerve, which has sympathetic fibers, to form the vidian nerve (**Fig. 6**). The vidian nerve delivers autonomic activity to the sphenopalatine ganglion and synapse with the postganglionic neurons before innervating the nasal mucosa.

### Inflammatory Pathway of Nose

The immune system in the nose is important to identify and combat inhaled foreign particles, such as allergens, toxins, and microbes. The complex immune responses are mediated by an innate and adaptive immunity.[24] Innate immunity acts as a nonspecific first-line defense against pathogens that are new to the host. This defense is made up of neutrophils, monocytes, mast cells, dendritic cells, and eosinophils. Working together, they eliminate infection through the activation of the complement system, natural killer cells, and toll-like receptor pathways. The adaptive immune

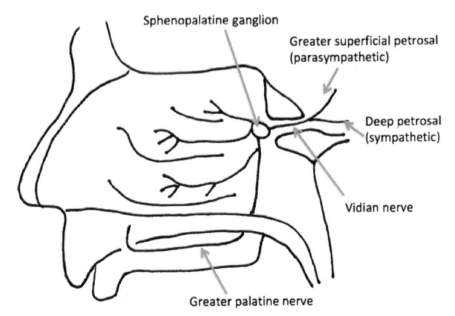

**Fig. 6.** Autonomic innervation of the nasal cavity.

response provides specificity and memory in fighting off pathogens through immunoglobulin and T-cell activity.

Allergens play a crucial role in the pathogenesis of aberrant inflammatory responses in the nose, which manifests as acute and chronic rhinosinusitis with nasal polyps. Allergens cause an immediate immunoglobulin E (IgE) hypersensitivity response, also known as type 1 hypersensitivity.[24] Early responses include mast cell degranulation and releases of histamine and proteases to cause vasodilation and glandular stimulation. Late responses include cytokine-mediated influx of eosinophils and activation of TH2 cells. Ultimately, this causes nasal congestion and rhinorrhea.

For medical therapy to mitigate the nasal inflammatory response and to reduce symptoms such as nasal obstruction, the AAO-HNS strongly recommends intranasal glucocorticosteroids and second-generation oral antihistamine drugs as first-line therapies.[25] Intranasal antihistamines are an option, especially in combination with intranasal steroids. Oral leukotriene receptor antagonists are not recommended as primary treatment.[25] Other therapies include decongestants, nasal irrigations, intranasal anticholinergics, or cromolyn sodium.

## Sinonasal Inflammatory Disease

Rhinitis refers to a heterogeneous group of nasal disorders characterized by symptoms of sneezing, nasal itching, rhinorrhea, and nasal congestion.[26,27] Rhinitis is divided into 2 major categories: allergic rhinitis (AR) and nonallergic rhinitis (NAR). AR is defined as a symptomatic nasal disorder mediated by IgE-mediated immune responses.[25] AR is one of the most common medical conditions affecting adults and is estimated to affect 1 in 6 Americans.[25] On the other hand, NAR is a non–IgE-mediated inflammatory response composed of a heterogeneous group of medical conditions. Like AR, it does significantly affect the quality of life of patients and is a clinical challenge. NAR has various forms, such as vasomotor rhinitis, infectious rhinitis, rhinitis due to hormonal changes, rhinitis from medications, or rhinitis due to systemic disease.

As described earlier, mucosal inflammation of the entire nasal cavity, but most importantly, inferior turbinate hypertrophy, occurs in these conditions due to inflammation, vascular dilation, and/or autonomic dysfunction. Furthermore, decreases in cross-sectional nasal area may have a more profound effect in patients with chronic rhinitis. They may experience more nasal resistance in certain positions such as supine or lateral decubitus positions due to higher sensitivities to changes in mucosal hydrostatic pressures or autonomic reflexes.[14]

Nasal obstruction is a hallmark symptom for sinusitis due to the presence of mucosal edema, purulence, and/or nasal polyposis. The impact on nasal airflow is three-fold[1]: anatomic blockage of normal airflow,[2] disruption of MCT, and[3] airflow receptor anomalies. Furthermore, the blockage of natural sinus drainage pathways and mucosal inflammation exacerbate the feeling of nasal congestion.

## Iatrogenic Causes of Nasal Obstruction

Iatrogenic causes of nasal obstruction may arise after nasal and sinus surgery. Adhesions and synechia formation are among common minor complications of endoscopic sinus surgery.[28,29] In rhinoplasty, failure to reconnect the ULCs to the septum causes inferior-medial collapse of the ULCs, the pinching of the middle vault, and internal valve airflow obstruction. Other causes of iatrogenic nasal obstruction in rhinoplasty are overresection of lower lateral crura to reduce external nasal valve strength and aberrant osteotomies that may cause collapse of nasal bones.

## SUMMARY

Nasal obstruction is a common presenting symptom to both primary care physicians and otolaryngologists. Causes of nasal obstruction may be isolated but are more likely multifactorial. Understanding the anatomy and physiology of nasal obstruction is crucial for optimal diagnosis and management.

## REFERENCES

1. Fettman N, Sanford T, Sindwani R. Surgical management of the deviated septum: techniques in septoplasty. Otolaryngologic Clin North America 2009;42(2): 241–52.
2. Keeler J, Most SP. Measuring nasal obstruction. Facial Plast Surg Clin North America 2016;24(3):315–22.
3. Franciscus RG, Trinkaus E. Nasal morphology and the emergence of Homo erectus. Am J Phys Anthropol 1988;75(4):517–27.
4. Sozansky J, Houser SM. The physiological mechanism for sensing nasal airflow: a literature review. Int Forum Allergy Rhinology 2014;4(10):834–8.
5. Numa W, Johnson C. Surgical anatomy and physiology of the nose. Master techniques in rhinoplasty. Philadelphia: Elsevier; 2011. p. 21–30.
6. Becker D, Guyuron B. Nasal reconstruction and aesthetic rhinoplasty. In: Siemionow MZ, Eisenmann-Klein M, editors. Plastic and Reconstructive Surgery. Springer Specialist Surgery Series. London: Springer; 2010.
7. Ferril GR, Winkler AA. Rhinoplasty and nasal reconstruction. In: Scholes MA, Ramakrishnan VR, editors. ENT secrets. Philadelphia: Elsevier; 2016. p. 405–11.
8. Holt GR. Biomechanics of nasal septal trauma. Otolaryngol Clin North Am 1999; 32(4):615–9.
9. Costa DJ, Sanford T, Janney C, et al. Radiographic and anatomic characterization of the nasal septal swell body. Arch Otolaryngology–Head Neck Surg 2010;136(11):1107.
10. Wexler D, Braverman M. Histology of the nasal septal swell body (septal turbinate). Otolaryngol Head Neck Surg 2006;134(4):596–600.
11. Jourdy D. Inferior turbinate reduction. Oper Tech Otolaryngology-Head Neck Surg 2014;25(2):160–70.
12. Berger G, Balum-Azim M, Ophir D. The normal inferior turbinate: histomorphometric analysis and clinical implications. The Laryngoscope 2003;113(7):1192–8.
13. Peric A, Sotirovic J, Baletic N, et al. Concha bullosa and the nasal middle meatus obstructive syndrome. Vojnosanit Pregl 2008;65(3):255–8.
14. Chandra RK, Patadia MO, Raviv J. Diagnosis of nasal airway obstruction. Otolaryngologic Clin North America 2009;42(2):207–25.
15. Rhee JS, Weaver EM, Park SS, et al. Clinical consensus statement: diagnosis and management of nasal valve compromise. Otolaryngology-Head Neck Surg 2010; 143(1):48–59.
16. Osborn JL, Sacks R. Chapter 2: nasal obstruction. Am J Rhinology Allergy 2013; 27(3):7–8.
17. Ramsden JD, Campisi P, Forte V. Choanal atresia and choanal stenosis. Otolaryngologic Clin North America 2009;42(2):339–52.
18. Stamm AC, Shirley SN, Balsalobre L. Transnasal endoscopic-assisted surgery of the anterior skull base. In: Flint PW, Haughey BH, Lund V, et al, editors. Cummings otolaryngology. Philadelphia: Saunders; 2015. p. 2701–18.
19. Simmen DB, Jones NS. Epistaxis. In: Flint PW, Haughey BH, Lund V, et al, editors. Cummings otolaryngology. Philadelphia: Saunders; 2015. p. 678–90.

20. Chegar BE, Tatum SA. Nasal fractures. In: Flint PW, Haughey BH, Lund V, et al, editors. Cummings otolaryngology. Philadelphia: Saunders; 2015. p. 493–505.
21. Pallanch J, Jorissen M. Objective assessment of nasal function. In: Flint PW, Haughey BH, Lund V, et al, editors. Cummings otolaryngology. Philadelphia: Saunders; 2015. p. 644–57.
22. Kahana-Zweig R, Geva-Sagiv M, Weissbrod A, et al. Measuring and characterizing the human nasal cycle. PLoS One 2016;11(10):e0162918.
23. Kridel R, Sturm-O'brien A. Nasal septum. In: Flint PW, Haughey BH, Lund V, et al, editors. Cummings otolaryngology. Philadelphia: Saunders; 2015. p. 474–92.
24. Baroody FM, Naclerio RM. Allergy and immunology of the upper airway. In: Flint PW, Haughey BH, Lund V, et al, editors. Cummings otolaryngology. Philadelphia: Saunders; 2015. p. 593–625.
25. Seidman MD, Gurgel RK, Lin SY, et al. Clinical practice guideline: allergic rhinitis. Otolaryngol Head Neck Surg 2015;152(1 Suppl):S1–43.
26. Wallace D, Dykewicz M, Bernstein D, et al. The diagnosis and management of rhinitis: an updated practice parameter. J Allergy Clin Immunol 2008;122(2): S1–84.
27. Orlandi RR, Kingdom TT, Hwang PH, et al. International consensus statement on allergy and rhinology: rhinosinusitis. Int Forum Allergy Rhinology 2016;6(S1): S22–209.
28. Bhatiki AM, Goldberg AN. Complications of surgery of the paranasal sinuses. In: Eisele DW, Smith RV, editors. Complications in head and neck surgery. Philadelphia: Mosby; 2009. p. 543–58.
29. Kim DW, Jafer Ali M. Complications of rhinoplasty. In: Eisele DW, Smith RV, editors. Complications in head and neck surgery. Philadelphia: Mosby; 2009. p. 559–76.

# Diagnostic Algorithm for Evaluating Nasal Airway Obstruction

Jennifer A. Villwock, MD[a],*, Ronald B. Kuppersmith, MD[b]

## KEYWORDS

- Nasal obstruction • Diagnosis • Cause • Examination

## KEY POINTS

- Nasal airway obstruction is a common complaint with multiple possible causes.
- A thorough evaluation of patient history and nasal anatomy is necessary for establishing an accurate diagnosis and initiating appropriate and targeted intervention.
- A diagnostic algorithm can aid in the development of a systematic approach to nasal obstruction evaluation and selection of treatment options.

Nasal airway obstruction (NAO) is a common symptom that significantly impairs quality of life. It also can be challenging for clinicians to treat because the severity of nasal obstruction is typically subjective and does not necessarily correlate to an objective examination or test. Although validated instruments, such as the Nasal Obstruction and Septoplasty Effectiveness Scale (NOSE), can be used to help clinicians and patients better communicate about the severity of symptoms, they do not help clinicians accurately identify the underlying cause.[1,2] Additionally, by the time patients present for evaluation, they have tried numerous different treatments and think that their symptoms are severe and unmanageable enough that further help is needed.

Effective treatment of NAO requires an accurate diagnosis. There is no single test that correlates specifically to the underlying cause of NAO in all patients. It is essential for the clinician to evaluate patients in a systematic fashion. Identification of all

Disclosure Statement: R.B. Kuppersmith is a consultant for Entellus Medical and Arrinex. J.A. Villwock has nothing to disclose.
[a] Department of Otolaryngology, Head and Neck Surgery, University of Kansas Medical Center, Kansas University, 3901 Rainbow Boulevard, MS 3010, Kansas City, KS 66160, USA;
[b] Department of Surgery, Texas A&M Health Science Center, 1730 Birmingham Drive, College Station, TX 77845, USA
* Corresponding author.
E-mail address: jvillwock@kumc.edu

Otolaryngol Clin N Am 51 (2018) 867–872
https://doi.org/10.1016/j.otc.2018.05.002
0030-6665/18/© 2018 Elsevier Inc. All rights reserved.

possible causes allows the clinician to appropriately tailor treatment plans. Treatment options may involve lifestyle changes, medications, and/or surgical intervention.

The underlying causes of NAO can be anatomic, related to normal physiology, or have a pathophysiologic basis. Furthermore, NAO can be static in nature and present all of the time or may be dynamic, fluctuating with respiratory effort, time, or other factors.[1,3,4] There are multiple potential causes for NAO in the differential diagnosis (**Fig. 1**, **Box 1**). It is also important to recognize that patient symptomatology may be multifactorial.

A thorough history and physical examination is the most important tool to delineate the underlying causes in a specific case. Nasal endoscopy, imaging, allergy testing, and other ancillary tests are tools that can be useful in evaluating these patients.

## HISTORY

When patients present with NAO, a thorough history is essential. Historical elements that should be considered include location of the obstruction; severity; elements of timing; the setting in which it occurs; aggravating factors; relieving factors; associated manifestations; previous testing; and response to previous treatments[3,5] (**Table 1**). Response or nonresponse to previous treatments can provide diagnostic clues.

## PHYSICAL EXAMINATION

The physical examination is equally crucial to narrowing the differential diagnosis and establishing the correct diagnosis. An important component of the physical examination begins with the history taking. *Observation* of patients during this time is essential.

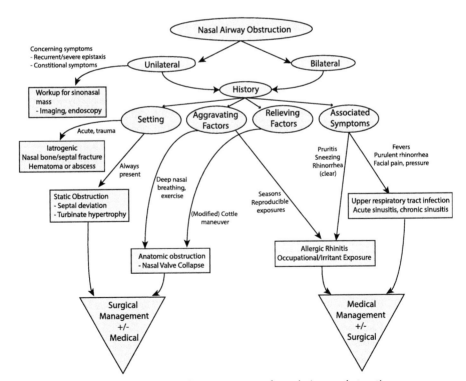

**Fig. 1.** Algorithm to evaluation and management of nasal airway obstruction.

---

**Box 1**
**Differential diagnosis of nasal airway obstruction**

Anatomic
  Septal deviation
  Turbinate hypertrophy
  Concha bullosa
  Lateral nasal wall
  Adenoid hypertrophy

Physiologic
  Nasal cycle
  Pregnancy

Pathophysiologic
  Inflammatory/mucosal
    Allergic
    Infectious (viral, bacterial, fungal)
    Nasal polyps
    Granulomatous
  Vasomotor/neurogenic
  External stimuli
    Rhinitis medicamentosa
    Alcohol
    Cigarettes
    Other medications
  Congenital
    Choanal atresia
  Iatrogenic/traumatic
    Septal perforation
    Septal hematoma
    Septal abscess
    Foreign body
  Neoplasm
    Juvenile nasopharyngeal angiofibroma
    Inverted papilloma
    Squamous cell carcinoma
    Other malignancy
  Metabolic
    Hypothyroidism

---

A basic NAO *physical examination* includes, at a minimum, a head and neck examination, including anterior rhinoscopy and maneuvers like the Cottle and modified Cottle, and endoscopy.[6]

*Anterior rhinoscopy* should be performed, ideally with a bright light and a nasal speculum with patients sitting upright. In children, and when a nasal speculum is not available, a handheld otoscope can be used to perform anterior rhinoscopy.[5] If the nasopharynx, posterior aspect of the septum, middle turbinate, and middle meatus are visible, these should be evaluated as well. If the patients' septum is deviated, it should be noted if the deviation correlates with the description of the patients' symptoms. For example, if the septum is deviated to the left, and patients describe left-sided obstruction, then the septum is a likely contributor to their symptoms. However, it is important to keep in mind that the septum can have multiple areas of deformity. The septum can be S shaped, have accordion-type fractures with multiple points of deviation, or have simple spurs that obstruct both sides.[7,8]

The location and mucosa of the inferior turbinates should be carefully noted. Enlarged inferior turbinates, which project into the nasal cavity and/or contact the

| Table 1<br>Elements to consider in patient history for nasal airway obstruction | |
|---|---|
| Location | • Is it unilateral or bilateral obstruction?<br>• If it is unilateral, which side is it?<br>• If it is bilateral, is either side worse?<br>• Does obstruction fluctuate from side to side? |
| Severity | • Is it mild, moderate, severe, or very severe?<br>• Does it impact their ability to perform daily activities or exercise?<br>• Does the severity fluctuate?<br>• What is the NOSE score? |
| Timing | • How long has it been present?<br>• When did it start?<br>  ○ Are there any clear inciting events, trauma, and so forth?<br>• Is it constant or are there certain times of day or seasons of year that it is worse?<br>• Does it recur? |
| Setting | • Was there a specific location when it first occurred?<br>• Are there any new medications?<br>• Are they pregnant?<br>• Are there any recent sino-nasal or upper respiratory infections?<br>• Is there any exposure to chemical/occupational irritants? |
| Aggravating factors | • Does it occur inside vs outside?<br>• Do cigarettes or drinking alcohol make it worse?<br>• Is it made worse by eating spicy foods, lying down, dust/mold/pollen, temperature changes, and/or weather changes?<br>• Is it made worse by strong odors or fumes?<br>• Is it made worse by their work environment; if so, what is in the work environment? |
| Relieving factors | • Are there physical maneuvers, such as pulling the nose up, that relieve it?<br>• Does elevating the head or use of nasal strips or cones help? |
| Associated manifestations | • Allergic/irritant<br>  ○ Eye pruritis<br>  ○ Nasal pruritis<br>  ○ Frequent sneezing<br>  ○ Cough<br>• Infectious<br>  ○ Fevers<br>  ○ Facial pain/pressure<br>  ○ Purulent drainage<br>  ○ Sinusitis<br>• Miscellaneous<br>  ○ Cough<br>  ○ Postnasal drainage<br>  ○ Snoring<br>  ○ Popping or pressure in the ears<br>  ○ Olfactory or gustatory dysfunction<br>  ○ Epistaxis |

septum, can be a significant cause of nasal obstruction. This condition can be caused by an allergy, the nasal cycle, and/or other inflammatory causes.[9] Additionally, if the septum is severely deviated to one side, the inferior turbinate on the contralateral side can be very hypertrophic.[10]

A *modified Cottle maneuver* should be performed. Patients should be instructed to breathe through their nose gently and then with maximal nasal inspiration. The lateral nasal wall, ala, and vestibule are observed for signs of collapse or dynamic obstruction. Patients are asked if the exaggerated nasal breathing impacts their nasal obstruction. A cotton swab or cerumen loop can then be placed through the nasal vestibule to support the lateral wall cartilage to see if this provides improvement in their airway.[6] If they have improvement with this maneuver, nasal valve collapse is a source of their nasal obstruction. The *Cottle maneuver* can also be performed by placing 1 or 2 fingertips on the cheek adjacent to the nasal sidewall and then applying gentle lateral traction. Improvement with the Cottle maneuver also implicates the internal nasal valve as a source of obstruction.[6,11]

To observe the impact of topical decongestion on intranasal topography, *topical decongestant* can then be sprayed into the patients' nose. If patients frequently use these topical decongestants, it may not have the desired effect. Similarly, if there is inferior turbinate hypertrophy that is primarily bony in nature, decongestion may not have a significant impact on the nasal airway. The physician should wait several minutes for the decongestant to work. Patients should be asked if they notice improvement; if they do, this suggests an underlying inflammatory cause and, frequently, prominent submucosal turbinate hypertrophy. Anterior rhinoscopy and the modified Cottle maneuver should be repeated to determine if decongestion changes the appearance of the inferior turbinates, reveals a deeper view into the nasal cavity, or affects the efficacy of the modified Cottle maneuver.

*Nasal endoscopy*, although not essential in every case, permits a detailed evaluation of the entire nasal cavity and nasopharynx. This information can be particularly helpful to evaluate the posterior aspect of the nasal cavity and nasopharynx, to see past significant anterior obstruction, to evaluate the status of the adenoid, and to look for pathologic masses. It also allows for the evaluation of the middle turbinate, middle meatus, and sphenoethmoid recess for evidence of inflammation or other signs of sinus disease that might otherwise be missed. For example, polypoid change of the middle turbinate, an entity distinct from nasal polyposis and associated with concomitant uncontrolled allergy, may become apparent and help guide more aggressive allergy management in addition to other measures.[12] Typically, multiple passes are recommended to allow complete visualization of the inferior turbinate and inferior meatus; the middle turbinate and middle meatus; and the sphenoethmoid recess, choana, and nasopharynx.

*Sinus imaging,* in particular maxillofacial computed tomography without contrast, can be helpful to evaluate nasal polyps, other pathologic masses, and to determine the presence of a concha bullosa or other anatomic variations that may contribute to nasal obstruction. Additional imaging can be considered if there are concerning findings on examination or imaging.

*Ancillary tests*, such as *allergy testing*, can be helpful to evaluate for underlying causes of allergic rhinitis and to facilitate immunotherapy.[13] Other tests that might be helpful in selected cases include *olfactory testing, MRI, clinical photographs,* and *laboratory evaluation.*[14]

## SUMMARY

There may be multiple causes to nasal obstruction in a specific patient. A systematic approach to ensure correct diagnoses of all contributing factors is essential for successful treatment. This approach allows the clinician to estimate the contribution of each factor and determine how aggressive each underlying cause should be addressed to help alleviate the symptoms.

**REFERENCES**

1. Haye R, Døsen LK, Tarangen M, et al. Good correlation between visual analogue scale and numerical rating scale in the assessment of nasal obstruction. J Laryngol Otol 2018;132(4):327–8.
2. Lodder WL, Leong SC. What are the clinically important outcome measures in the surgical management of nasal obstruction? Clin Otolaryngol 2018;43(2):567–71.
3. Esmaili A, Acharya A. Clinical assessment, diagnosis and management of nasal obstruction. Aust Fam Physician 2017;46(7):499–503.
4. Teichgraeber JF, Gruber RP, Tanna N. Surgical management of nasal airway obstruction. Clin Plast Surg 2016;43(1):41–6.
5. Kohlberg GD, Stewart MG, Ward RF, et al. Evaluation and management of pediatric nasal obstruction: a survey of practice patterns. Am J Rhinol Allergy 2016; 30(4):274–8.
6. Fung E, Hong P, Moore C, et al. The effectiveness of modified cottle maneuver in predicting outcomes in functional rhinoplasty. Plast Surg Int 2014;2014:618313.
7. Garcia GJM, Rhee JS, Senior BA, et al. Septal deviation and nasal resistance: an investigation using virtual surgery and computational fluid dynamics. Am J Rhinol Allergy 2010;24(1):e46–53.
8. Mariño-Sánchez F, Valls-Mateus M, Cardenas-Escalante P, et al. Influence of nasal septum deformity on nasal obstruction, disease severity, and medical treatment response among children and adolescents with persistent allergic rhinitis. Int J Pediatr Otorhinolaryngol 2017;95:145–54.
9. Sharhan SSA, Lee EJ, Hwang CS, et al. Radiological comparison of inferior turbinate hypertrophy between allergic and non-allergic rhinitis: does allergy really augment turbinate hypertrophy? Eur Arch Otorhinolaryngol 2018;275(4):923–9.
10. Chiesa Estomba C, Rivera Schmitz T, Ossa Echeverri CC, et al. Compensatory hypertrophy of the contralateral inferior turbinate in patients with unilateral nasal septal deviation. A computed tomography study. Otolaryngol Pol 2015;69(2): 14–20.
11. Fedok FG. Update in the management of the middle vault in rhinoplasty. Curr Opin Otolaryngol Head Neck Surg 2016;24(4):279–84.
12. Brunner JP, Jawad BA, McCoul ED. Polypoid change of the middle turbinate and paranasal sinus polyposis are distinct entities. Otolaryngol Head Neck Surg 2017;157(3):519–23.
13. Seidman MD, Gurgel RK, Lin SY, et al. Clinical practice guideline: allergic rhinitis. Otolaryngol Head Neck Surg 2015;152(1 Suppl):S1–43.
14. Banglawala SM, Oyer SL, Lohia S, et al. Olfactory outcomes in chronic rhinosinusitis with nasal polyposis after medical treatments: a systematic review and meta-analysis. Int Forum Allergy Rhinol 2014;4(12):986–94.

# Treatment Paradigm for Nasal Airway Obstruction

Theodore A. Schuman, MD[a], Brent A. Senior, MD[b],*

## KEYWORDS

- Nasal airway obstruction • Treatment • Septal deviation • Internal nasal valve
- External nasal valve • Nasal turbinate

## KEY POINTS

- Pathology leading to symptomatic nasal obstruction may be structural, inflammatory, or other in nature; most patients have more than 1 factor contributing to persistent nasal congestion.
- Medical therapy for nasal obstruction focuses on controlling inflammatory mucosal disease.
- Optimizing outcomes in surgery for nasal airway obstruction requires careful preoperative evaluation, including nasal endoscopy, to accurately identify contributing factors in individual patients.
- The internal nasal valve has the narrowest cross-sectional area within the nasal airway and is thus most sensitive to changes in its dimension due to anatomic variation or surgical intervention.

## INTRODUCTION

Nasal airway obstruction (NAO) is a common otolaryngic complaint, with estimates of up to one-third of the adult population having some degree of NAO and one-quarter of affected patients seeking intervention.[1] An estimated 9.5 million office visits occurred in the United States in 2006 for the evaluation of nasal congestion.[2] The monetary cost of nasal obstruction is significant. Approximately 3 decades ago, Kimmelman[3] estimated $5 billion were spent annually for symptomatic relief and another $60 million on surgical procedures to address anatomic causes of obstruction. Surgical intervention to alleviate recalcitrant nasal blockage is commonly performed both in the United States[4] and in other developed countries.[5]

Disclosure Statement: Dr B.A. Senior is an unpaid consultant to Spirox.
[a] Rhinology, Allergy, and Skull Base Surgery, Department of Otolaryngology–Head and Neck Surgery, Virginia Commonwealth University, 1200 East Broad Street, Suite 12-313, PO Box 980146, Richmond, VA 23298, USA; [b] Division of Rhinology, Allergy, and Skull Base Surgery, Department of Otolaryngology–Head and Neck Surgery, University of North Carolina at Chapel Hill, 170 Manning Drive, CB #7070, Chapel Hill, NC 27599-7070, USA
* Corresponding author.
E-mail address: brent_senior@med.unc.edu

Otolaryngol Clin N Am 51 (2018) 873–882
https://doi.org/10.1016/j.otc.2018.05.003
0030-6665/18/© 2018 Elsevier Inc. All rights reserved.

oto.theclinics.com

The anatomy and physiology of nasal airflow are complex subjects addressed in greater detail in, David W. Hsu and Jeffrey D. Suh's article, "Anatomy and Physiology of Nasal Obstruction," in this issue. The rigid framework supporting the nasal airway is provided by the bony and cartilaginous septum and paired nasal bones. The bony septum consists of the vomer, perpendicular plate of the ethmoid, and maxillary crest. The lateral nasal walls contain the paired inferior, middle, and superior turbinates, sometimes supplemented by the supreme turbinates. The turbinates have both bony and soft tissue components and thus may represent both fixed and variable sources of nasal obstruction. The internal nasal valve is formed by the nasal septum, upper lateral cartilage (ULC), and head of the inferior turbinate and is the region of the nose with the narrowest cross-sectional area. The normal angle between the nasal septum and ULC is 10° to 15°; small decreases in this angle may result in symptoms of nasal blockage.[6] The external nasal valve is caudal to the internal valve and represents the soft tissues of the nasal vestibule, consisting of the septum, columella, nasal sill, and ala[7] (**Fig. 1**). The posterior limit of the nasal cavity is delineated by the choanae, which serve as the transition point to the nasopharynx.

The velocity of nasal airflow is inversely related to the cross-sectional area within a particular subsite of the nasal airway; the internal nasal valve has the smallest area and thus the most rapid airflow. Bernoulli's law dictates that an increase in velocity is associated with a decrease in intraluminal pressure. The resulting pressure differential induces a collapse of surrounding soft tissue and worsening of airway obstruction. Furthermore, Poiseuille's law explains that the flow of a fluid, in this case air through the nasal cavity, is inversely proportional to the fourth power of the radius of the lumen. As a result, even small modifications to the cross-sectional area of the nasal airway can produce dramatic effects on airflow, particularly through the internal nasal valve.[5]

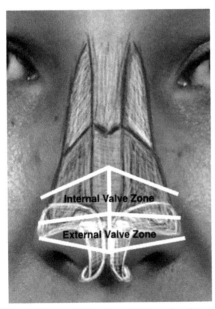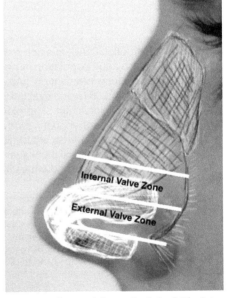

**Fig. 1.** Zones of lateral nasal sidewall collapse (left: coronal view; right: sagittal view). The internal valve zone corresponds to the inferior portion of the ULC and scroll region. The external valve zone corresponds to the soft tissues of the nasal ala. (*From* Barrett DM, Casanueva FJ, Cook TA. Management of the nasal valve. Facial Plast Surg Clin N Am 2016;24(3):221; with permission.)

Nasal valve collapse is a common finding, estimated to be an etiologic factor in 13% of adults with chronic nasal obstruction[8] and up to 95% of patients with persistent nasal congestion after septoplasty.[9]

Evaluation of patients with symptomatic NAO is addressed in detail in Jennifer Villwock and Ronald B. Kuppersmith's article, "Diagnostic Algorithm for Evaluating Nasal Airway Obstruction," in this issue. Several objective methods are available for measuring nasal airflow, including acoustic rhinometry, rhinomanometry, and peak inspiratory flow. Correlation of objective results with subjective symptoms is imperfect[6,10–12] and routine clinical use of such objective measures is not commonplace. Evaluation of airway obstruction typically centers around a patient's symptoms, which can be expressed subjectively or measured using validated instruments, such as the Nasal Obstruction Symptom Evaluation (NOSE) questionnaire.[13] Although clinically useful, the NOSE score has not been demonstrated to correlate with objective measurements of nasal airflow.[14]

Subtle variations in nasal anatomy at multiple levels can contribute to symptomatic nasal obstruction. Due to the previously described geometry of this area, impingement on the internal nasal valve typically has the greatest effect on nasal airflow. Sources contributing to NAO are listed in **Table 1** and are divided into structural, inflammatory, and other etiologies. It is important to recognize that multiple sources of nasal obstruction often exist within a given patient and that not all etiologies are appropriately

**Table 1**
**Factors contributing to symptomatic nasal obstruction**

| Structural | Inflammatory | Other |
|---|---|---|
| NSD | Chronic rhinitis | Atrophic rhinitis/ENS |
|   Body |   Allergic | Rhinitis medicamentosa |
|   Caudal septum |   Nonallergic | Other medications |
| Inferior turbinate hypertrophy |   Occupational |   (propranolol, |
|   Bony | Chronic rhinosinusitis |   chlorpromazine, |
|   Mucosal |   Without polyposis |   reserpine) |
| Middle turbinate hypertrophy/ |   With polyposis | Pregnancy |
|   concha bullosa |     Allergic fungal sinusitis | |
| Internal nasal valve abnormality | Tobacco use | |
|   Narrowing | Autoimmune disease | |
|   Dynamic collapse |   ANCA-associated | |
| External nasal valve/nasal |     Vasculitis/granulomatosis | |
|   vestibule abnormality |     With polyangiitis | |
|   Narrowing |   Sarcoidosis | |
|   Dynamic collapse |   Eosinophilic granulomatosis | |
| Intranasal mass |     With polyangiitis (Churg- | |
|   Inflammatory polyp |     Strauss syndrome) | |
|   Neoplasm | Other infectious | |
|   Congenital mass |   Vestibulitis | |
| Other septal pathology |   Rhinosporidiosis | |
|   Perforation |   Rhinoscleroma | |
|   Synechiae |   Adenoiditis | |
| Trauma | Gastroesophageal reflux | |
|   Deformity of nasal bones |   disease | |
|   Septal hematoma | Ciliary dysfunction | |
| |   Cystic fibrosis | |
| |   Primary ciliary dyskinesia | |

Blockage of nasal airflow may have structural, inflammatory, or other contributions and typically multiple etiologies are present within a given patient.

addressed via surgical intervention. Preoperative nasal endoscopy in the clinic setting is a critical component of evaluation of the patient with rhinologic complaints and may identify inflammatory or neoplastic disease not appreciated via anterior rhinoscopy.

## DISCUSSION

A systematic approach to managing the patient with nasal obstruction is delineated later. This paradigm is tailored to individual patients based on a complete rhinologic evaluation, including detailed history and nasal endoscopy, the latter of which is critical to accurately identifying specific sites of pathology as well as the presence of coexistent inflammatory disease. A careful patient history is mandatory and may suggest a contributing etiology and potential treatment. For example, chronic use of topical nasal decongestant resulting in significant rebound congestion (rhinitis medicamentosa) can be treated with discontinuation of the offending agent and the addition of topical and/or systemic steroids. Certain oral medications may also induce symptoms of chronic nasal congestion, as may pregnancy.[15] Components of the history and physical examination with particular relevance to the work-up of the patient with nasal obstruction are listed in **Table 2**.

**Table 2**
**Components of the history and physical examination that may aid in identification of etiologies of nasal obstruction**

| History | Physical Examination |
|---|---|
| Nature of nasal obstruction | Complete head and neck examination |
|   Unilateral vs bilateral |   Evidence of atopy (conjunctivitis, allergic shiners, |
|   Perennial vs seasonal |     supratip crease) |
|   Timing throughout day |   Evidence of malignancy (lymphadenopathy, |
|   Relation to environmental exposures |     cranial nerve |
|   Duration |   deficit) |
| Associated sinonasal symptoms | Nasal examination |
|   Hyposmia/anosmia |   External examination (nasal deformity, dynamic |
|   Nasal discharge (purulent vs other) |     collapse of nasal sidewall) |
|   Facial pain/pressure |   Anterior rhinoscopy (inferior turbinates, septum, |
| Other atopic symptoms |     internal nasal valve, evidence of inflammation) |
|   Sneezing |   Modified Cottle maneuver |
|   Itchy, watery eyes | Nasal endoscopy |
|   Eczema |   Septal deviation |
|   Asthma |   Turbinate enlargement |
|   Food allergy |   Mass or polyp |
|   Known environmental triggers |   Mucosal edema |
| History of sinonasal surgery or trauma |   Discharge |
| Medications |   Scarring |
|   Topical |   Crusting |
|   Systemic |   Dynamic collapse of internal valve |
| Social history |   Foreign body |
|   Tobacco use |   Adenoid enlargement |
|   Illicit intranasal drug use | |
|   Work/occupational exposures | |
| Pregnancy | |

Anterior rhinoscopy and nasal endoscopy may be performed before and after application of topical decongestant to assess the contribution of reversible mucosal edema to symptoms of blockage.

*Data from* Teichgraeber JF, Gruber RP, Tanna N. Surgical management of nasal airway obstruction. Clin Plast Surg 2016;43(1):41–6; and Osborn JL, Sacks R. Chapter 2: nasal obstruction. Am J Rhinol Allergy 2013;27(Suppl 1):7–8.

Nasal endoscopy may reveal evidence of significant mucosal inflammation, including edema, polyps, crusting, and rhinorrhea. Although numerous local and systemic pathologies can lead to inflammation of the upper airway, those seen most commonly in the otolaryngic practice include chronic rhinosinusitis with or without nasal polyposis, allergic or nonallergic rhinitis, and direct effects of irritants, such as tobacco smoke or occupational exposures. Less commonly, autoimmune disorders, such as granulomatosis with polyangiitis/antineutrophil cytoplasmic antibodies (ANCA)-associated vasculitis or sarcoidosis can cause chronic mucosal inflammation and crusting that significantly impair nasal airflow.[16]

In patients with substantial endoscopic evidence of mucosal inflammation, symptoms of nasal congestion or blockage may fluctuate, and careful history taking may reveal a pattern of symptoms suggestive of a specific culprit, such as environmental allergy or occupational exposure. Additional physical examination findings—presence of supratip crease, allergic shiners, and allergic conjunctivitis—may support the diagnosis of allergic rhinitis, which affects 10% to 30% of the adult population and up to 40% of children.[17] In these situations, aggressive management of allergies with topical and systemic therapies is appropriate. Consistent daily use of a nasal steroid spray is a typical first-line approach. Recalcitrant allergy symptoms may necessitate in vitro or skin allergy testing and consideration of sublingual or subcutaneous allergen immunotherapy. In patients with both distinct anatomic obstruction as well as chronic rhinitis, poor control of concurrent inflammatory disease may lead to suboptimal outcomes after surgery. Karatzanis and colleagues[18] reported that rhinomanometry improved to a significantly lesser degree in patients with concurrent allergic rhinitis and nasal septal deviation (NSD) treated with septoplasty, highlighting the need for ongoing medical management and careful counseling regarding patient expectations.

Other medical comorbidities may contribute to ongoing symptoms of nasal obstruction. Gastroesophageal reflux disease is typically associated with laryngopharyngeal symptoms, such as throat clearing and postnasal drip. It may play a significant role in nasal obstruction, however, particularly in children, who may note significant improvement in nasal congestion with antireflux therapy.[19] Cigarette smoking has been associated with reduced cross-sectional area of the nasal airway, diminished compliance, and lower peak inspiratory flow[20] as well as greater total nasal resistance when supine.[21] Counseling regarding smoking cessation and tempering expectations in the setting of ongoing tobacco dependence are critical in the preoperative setting.

Identification of a space-occupying lesion, such as inflammatory polyp, congenital mass, or neoplasm, necessitates management specific to the given pathology, discussion of which is beyond the scope of this article. The remainder of this discussion focuses on patients in whom mass lesions or significant inflammatory burden have been ruled out or appropriately treated. As noted in **Table 1**, anatomic variations at multiple nasal subsites can contribute to subjective nasal obstruction, and patients often have more than 1 etiology contributing to symptoms of nasal blockage. As such, it is common to perform multiple concurrent procedures to address distinct sites of obstruction.[22]

Preoperative evaluation focuses on identification of anatomic factors contributing to blockage of the nasal airway. Anterior rhinoscopy and nasal endoscopy are critical to diagnose common causes of NAO, such as inferior turbinate hypertrophy and NSD. **Fig. 2** demonstrates evaluation of the internal nasal valve via anterior rhinoscopy as well as through examination of nasal width through the oblique view.[23] The internal and external nasal valves should be visualized both statically and during inspiration to assess for dynamic collapse. A modified Cottle maneuver is helpful in diagnosing internal nasal valve collapse and simulating the effect of surgical widening of the angle

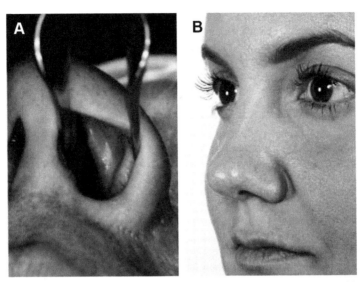

**Fig. 2.** (*A*) The internal nasal valve angle inside the nose. (*B*) The utility of the oblique view of the nose when examining the patient for internal nasal valve narrowing. (*From* Recker C, Hamilton GS. Evaluation of the patient with nasal obstruction. Facial Plast Surg 2016;32(1):4; with permission.)

between the nasal septum and ULC. This can be performed in clinic by assessing subjective nasal airflow before and after displacing the ULC laterally (for static collapse) or simple support of the ULC (for dynamic collapse), using a cotton swab or ear curette placed intranasally. Fung and colleagues[24] reported that the modified Cottle maneuver predicted symptomatic improvement after surgical intervention for internal nasal valve collapse, highlighting the clinical utility of this diagnostic technique.

Tsao and colleagues[25] proposed a system for quantification of lateral nasal wall collapse in which the nasal sidewall in divided into 2 zones: zone I is cephalad, at the level of the ULC/cartilaginous scroll, and zone II is caudad, at the level of the ala, the latter representing the traditional location of the external valve. The magnitude of dynamic collapse of the nasal sidewall is classified as grade 1 (<33%), grade 2 (33%–66%), or grade 3 (>66%).[14] This system may be useful in further classifying nasal valve collapse and predicting patients who would benefit from surgical intervention.

In patients with obvious nasal valve collapse/lateral nasal wall insufficiency and an absence of inflammatory pathology, an initial trial of nasal steroid was not recommended by an expert consensus.[6] Noninvasive options can be considered in these patients. For example, mechanical dilators, such as external nasal strips (eg, Breathe Right strips, GlaxoSmithKline, London, United Kingdom), internal nasal stents (eg, Max-Air Nose Cones, Sanostec, Beverly Farms, Massachusetts), nasal clips, and septal stimulators are commercially available options. A review of 33 mechanical devices found external nasal dilator strips and nasal clips of value in certain patients with nasal obstruction, thus they may be considered as initial management options.[26]

Numerous techniques have been described for the surgical correction of nasal valve collapse; this topic is addressed in greater detail in Sheena Samra and colleagues' article, "Surgical Management of Nasal Valve Collapse," in this issue.

The goal of nasal valve surgery is to relieve symptoms of nasal obstruction by increasing cross-sectional airway anatomy and supporting the lateral nasal wall and alar rim to resists dynamic collapse. Septoplasty and inferior turbinate reduction are effective in improving cross-sectional airway size but do not address a narrow internal nasal valve angle or tendency of the nasal sidewall to collapse. Interventions aimed at stenting the nasal sidewall are numerous and may involve the placement of spreader, alar batten, lateral crural strut, alar rim, and butterfly grafts as well as flaring sutures.[7] More recently, absorbable nasal sidewall implants have been described for the treatment of nasal valve collapse (Latera, Spirox, Redwood City, California); these have the potential advantage of being placed in clinic under local anesthesia. Initial data series suggest a majority of patients experience reduction in symptoms of nasal obstruction at 12 months after placement of the implant.[27] Further data are required to assess the long-term utility of these devices compared with well-established surgical therapies for valve collapse.

NSD has an estimated prevalence of up to 80% of the general adult population.[28] In fact, 90% of adults examined in an otolaryngology clinic setting are found to have NSD[29] and surgical management for NAO commonly includes repair of the deviated septum. Despite this ubiquity of NSD in the adult population, objective methods for determining the clinical relevance of septal deviation are lacking. Garcia and colleagues[30] used computational fluid dynamics to model nasal airflow based on anterior versus posterior NSD. In keeping with the theory that airway impingement within the more caudal region of the internal nasal valve produces the greatest effect on nasal obstruction, they reported that anterior septal deviation led to the largest increase in nasal resistance, whereas deviation was better tolerated in the posterior nasal cavity. Although many factors influence the decision of whether or not to perform surgery in a given patient, these data may be useful in helping the surgeon determine the clinical relevance of a particular septal deviation as well as predicting the likelihood that correction will result in symptom improvement.

Repair of the deviated nasal septum involves creation of a submucoperichondreal and submucoperiosteal flap. Subsequently, the deviated and obstructing portions of the quadrangular cartilage and septal bone are removed while simultaneously preserving adequate support for the soft tissues of the nose. Typically this involves preservation of an adequate L-strut of native cartilage and bone along the dorsal and causal aspects of the septum.

Numerous techniques for septoplasty have been described. Although traditionally performed with headlight and speculum under direct visualization, advances in endoscopic instrumentation and high-definition imaging have led to increased adoption of endoscopic septoplasty. A recent meta-analysis of 14 studies comparing open and endoscopic septoplasty found a significant improvement in postoperative nasal obstruction and headache as well as a significantly lower number of complications (mucosal tear, synechiae, hemorrhage, and persistent septal deviation) in the endoscopic group.[28]

Leitzen and colleagues[31,32] noted a correlation between inferior turbinate size and symptoms of nasal obstruction as measured with the NOSE instrument. Surgical reduction of the inferior turbinates to improve nasal congestion is typically performed after a trial of medical therapy. Several techniques have been described for inferior turbinate reduction and range from simple bony out-fracture to radiofrequency ablation to resection (using a variety of devices) of submucosal soft tissue to partial or total removal of the turbinate. Regardless of technique, turbinate reduction is associated with improvement in symptoms of nasal obstruction; thus, the choice of method for inferior turbinate reduction is often surgeon dependent.

A subset of patients may report NAO despite having widely patent airways on physical examination and/or normal objective measurements of nasal airflow. Commonly referred to as empty nose syndrome (ENS), the precise etiology of this symptom-atology has not been completely elucidated. It is likely related to an altered sensation of airflow through the nasal cavity, impaired thermoreception/chemoreception, and a lack of mucosal cooling in the overly patent airway.[33–35] ENS can be induced or exac-erbated by surgical attempts to widen the nasal airway, particularly with aggressive reduction of the inferior turbinates. It is highly challenging to treat, with recalcitrant symptoms and significant psychological comorbidity commonplace. The best treat-ment of ENS is prevention, through the use of conservative and mucosal-sparing sur-gical techniques, particularly with regard to the inferior turbinates. These paradoxic symptoms also occur in patients with atrophic rhinitis and may be accompanied by foul smell, crusting, bleeding, and superimposed infection. Options for the manage-ment of existing atrophic rhinitis or ENS include nasal saline lavages, antibiotics, mucosal hydration ointments, and psychological intervention. Surgical treatments have also been described to augment the nasal sidewall and reduce nasal airway vol-ume; long-term efficacy of these techniques are unknown.[36]

## SUMMARY

The anatomy and physiology of nasal airflow are complex, and symptomatic obstruc-tion of nasal airflow has many potential causes. Optimal management of the patient with NAO requires careful evaluation to accurately identify the sources of pathology contributing to symptoms within a given patient. Surgical options for treatment of NAO are multiple and should be carefully tailored to these findings. Diligent preoper-ative counseling is critical to create realistic patient expectations and ensure that the proper procedures are performed to alleviate appropriate symptoms.

## REFERENCES

1. Bateman N, Woolford T. Informed consent for septal surgery: the evidence-base. J Laryngol Otol 2003;117(3):186–9.
2. Cherry DK, Hing E, Woodwell DA, et al. National ambulatory medical care survey: 2006 summary. Natl Health Stat Report 2008;6(3):1–39.
3. Kimmelman CP. The problem of nasal obstruction. Otolaryngol Clin North Am 1989;22(2):253–64.
4. Bhattacharyya N. Ambulatory sinus and nasal surgery in the United States: de-mographics and perioperative outcomes. Laryngoscope 2010;120(3):635–8.
5. Wever CC. The nasal airway: a critical review. Facial Plast Surg 2016;32:17–21.
6. Rhee JS, Weaver EM, Park SS, et al. Clinical consensus statement: diagnosis and management of nasal valve compromise. Otolaryngol Head Neck Surg 2010; 143(1):48–59.
7. Barrett DM, Casanueva FJ, Cook TA. Management of the nasal valve. Facial Plast Surg Clin North Am 2016;24(3):219–34.
8. Elwany S, Thabet H. Obstruction of the nasal valve. J Laryngol Otol 1996;110(3): 221–4.
9. Chambers KJ, Horstkotte KA, Shanley K, et al. Evaluation of improvement in nasal obstruction following nasal valve correction in patients with a history of failed sep-toplasty. JAMA Facial Plast Surg 2015;17(5):347–50.
10. Ishii LE, Rhee JS. Are diagnostic tests useful for nasal valve compromise? Laryn-goscope 2013;123(1):7–8.
11. Cannon DE, Rhee JS. Evidence-based practice. functional rhinoplasty. Otolar-yngol Clin North Am 2012;45(5):1033–43.

12. Andrã© RF, Vuyk HD, Ahmed A, et al. Correlation between subjective and objective evaluation of the nasal airway. A systematic review of the highest level of evidence. Clin Otolaryngol 2009;34(6):518–25.

13. Lipan MJ, Most SP. Development of a severity classification system for subjective nasal obstruction. JAMA Facial Plast Surg 2013;15(5):358–61.

14. Keeler J, Most SP. Measuring nasal obstruction. Facial Plast Surg Clin North Am 2016;24(3):315–22.

15. Teichgraeber JF, Gruber RP, Tanna N. Surgical management of nasal airway obstruction. Clin Plast Surg 2016;43(1):41–6.

16. Kuan EC, Suh JD. Systemic and odontogenic etiologies in chronic rhinosinusitis. Otolaryngol Clin North Am 2017;50(1):95–111.

17. Wallace DV, Dykewicz MS, Bernstein DI, et al. The diagnosis and management of rhinitis: an updated practice parameter. J Allergy Clin Immunol 2008; 122(2 Suppl):1–84.

18. Karatzanis AD, Fragiadakis G, Moshandrea J, et al. Septoplasty outcome in patients with and without allergic rhinitis. Rhinology 2009;47(4):444–9.

19. Megale SRMCL, Scanavini ABA, Andrade EC, et al. Gastroesophageal reflux disease: its importance in ear, nose, and throat practice. Int J Pediatr Otorhinolaryngol 2006;70(1):81–8.

20. Kjaergaard T, Cvancarova M, Steinsvaag SK. Smoker's nose: structural and functional characteristics. Laryngoscope 2010;120(7):1475–80.

21. Stroud RH, Wright ST, Calhoun KH. Nocturnal nasal congestion and nasal resistance. Laryngoscope 1999;109(9):1450–3.

22. Rhee JS, Arganbright JM, McMullin BT, et al. Evidence supporting functional rhinoplasty or nasal valve repair: a 25-year systematic review. Otolaryngol Head Neck Surg 2008;139(1):10–20.

23. Recker C, Hamilton GS. Evaluation of the patient with nasal obstruction. Facial Plast Surg 2016;32:3–8.

24. Fung E, Hong P, Moore C, et al. The effectiveness of modified cottle maneuver in predicting outcomes in functional rhinoplasty. Plast Surg Int 2014;2014:1–6.

25. Tsao GJ, Fijalkowski N, Most SP. Validation of a grading system for lateral nasal wall insufficiency. Allergy Rhinol (Providence) 2013;4(2):66–8.

26. Kiyohara N, Badger C, Tjoa T, et al. A comparison of over-the-counter mechanical nasal dilators. JAMA Facial Plast Surg 2016;18(5):385.

27. Nicolo MS, Stelter K, Sadick H, et al. Absorbable implant to treat nasal valve collapse. Facial Plast Surg 2017;33(2):233–40.

28. Hong CJ, Monteiro E, Badhiwala J, et al. Open versus endoscopic septoplasty techniques: a systematic review and meta-analysis. Am J Rhinol Allergy 2016; 30(6):436–42.

29. Mladina R, Čujić E, Šubarić M, et al. Nasal septal deformities in ear, nose, and throat patients. An international study. Am J Otolaryngol 2008;29(2):75–82.

30. Garcia GJM, Rhee JS, Senior BA, et al. Septal deviation and nasal resistance: an investigation using virtual surgery and computational fluid dynamics. Am J Rhinol Allergy 2010;24(1). https://doi.org/10.2500/ajra.2010.24.3428.

31. Leitzen KP, Brietzke SE, Lindsay RW. Correlation between nasal anatomy and objective obstructive sleep apnea severity. Otolaryngol Head Neck Surg 2014; 150(2):325–31.

32. Brunworth J, Holmes J, Sindwani R. Inferior turbinate hypertrophy: review and graduated approach to surgical management. Am J Rhinol Allergy 2013;27(5): 411–5.

33. Sozansky J, Houser SM. Pathophysiology of empty nose syndrome. Laryngoscope 2015;125(1):70–4.

34. Kimbell JS, Frank DO, Laud P, et al. Changes in nasal airflow and heat transfer correlate with symptom improvement after surgery for nasal obstruction. J Biomech 2013;46(15):2634–43.

35. Sullivan CD, Garcia GJM, Frank-Ito DO, et al. Perception of better nasal patency correlates with increased mucosal cooling after surgery for nasal obstruction. Otolaryngol Head Neck Surg 2014;150(1):139–47.

36. Osborn JL, Sacks R. Chapter 2: nasal obstruction. Am J Rhinol Allergy 2013; 27(Suppl 1):7–8.

# Measuring Nasal Obstruction Outcomes

Emily Spataro, MD, Sam P. Most, MD*

## KEYWORDS

- Nasal obstruction • Objective and subjective outcomes measures
- Functional rhinoplasty • Nasal valve stenosis • Patient-reported outcomes measures

## KEY POINTS

- Methods of measuring nasal obstruction include anatomic, physiologic, and patient-reported outcome measures.
- Anatomic measures include acoustic rhinometry, imaging studies, and clinician-derived examination findings.
- Physiologic measures include rhinomanometry, nasal peak inspiratory flow, and computational fluid dynamics.
- Patient-reported outcome measures include subjective assessments of nasal obstruction and sinonasal symptomatology.
- Correlation between objective and subjective outcome measures is controversial, with expert opinion favoring the use of patient-reported outcome measures for rhinoplasty outcomes.

## INTRODUCTION

Measuring nasal obstruction outcomes is complex due to the multifaceted etiology of nasal obstruction. Causes include inflammatory diseases, anatomic obstruction, or a combination of both. Inflammatory etiologies include diagnoses such as allergic rhinitis, chronic rhinosinusitis, and nasal polyposis. Anatomic etiologies include septal deviation, inferior turbinate hypertrophy, and nasal valve compromise. Nasal valve compromise can be further subdivided into internal or external nasal valve compromise, as well as static obstruction or dynamic collapse.[1] Nasal obstruction also may be compounded by physiologic factors, such as the nasal cycle, or decreased airflow sensation, as with empty nose syndrome.[2]

Just as there are many causes of nasal obstruction, there are also many methods of measuring it. Anatomic measurements determine the structure, cross-sectional area,

Disclosure Statement: The authors have nothing to disclose.
Division of Facial Plastic and Reconstructive Surgery, Stanford University School of Medicine, 801 Welch Road, Stanford, CA 94305, USA
* Corresponding author.
E-mail address: smost@stanford.edu

Otolaryngol Clin N Am 51 (2018) 883–895
https://doi.org/10.1016/j.otc.2018.05.013
0030-6665/18/© 2018 Elsevier Inc. All rights reserved.

oto.theclinics.com

and volume of the nasal airway. Those discussed in this article include acoustic rhinometry, imaging, and clinician-derived outcomes. Physiologic measurements determine nasal resistance and airflow. Rhinomanometry, peak nasal inspiratory flow, and computational fluid dynamics are examples of these modalities. There are multiple patient-reported outcome measures (PROMs) specific for nasal obstruction.[3–5] Several studies have attempted to correlate these various subjective and objective outcome measures, but few show strong statistical correlations.[6]

Given the lack of correlation found between objective and subjective nasal obstruction outcome measures, expert opinion has focused on determining successful surgical outcomes based on PROMs. For example, in the nasal valve compromise clinical consensus statement, PROMs were recognized as valid indicators of successful intervention.[1] Likewise, the rhinoplasty clinical consensus statement also recommends incorporation of PROMs for rhinoplasty surgery assessment.[7] Thus, the development and use of relevant and validated PROMs to evaluate treatment of nasal airway obstruction is an important component of both nasal obstruction outcomes research and patient care. The goal of this review was to provide a summary of current nasal obstruction outcomes measures to guide clinical decision making and research.

## ANATOMIC OUTCOME MEASURES
### Acoustic Rhinometry

Acoustic rhinometry (AR) uses acoustic reflections to calculate the cross-sectional area of the nasal airway. The AR device transmits sound waves to a patient's nasal cavity, and then records the sound waves as they are reflected back. The amplitude of reflected sound waves correlates with changes in nasal airway cross-sectional area; the time between reflections is used to calculate the distance between these changes as a function of the longitudinal distance along the nasal passage.[8] These results can then be used to calculate the minimum cross-sectional area of the airway and the volume of the nasal passage.[9–12] AR has been validated against methods such as computed tomography (CT), MRI, and nasal endoscopy.[8,13–18] Advantages of AR include that it is fast, requires little instruction, and can be used in younger children.[19] Despite these advantages, limitations of AR include that it is a static measurement of nasal dimension, assumes that the nasal tissues are static and cannot measure dynamic changes with breathing, and does not take into account factors such as nasal congestion. Testing, therefore, should be conducted before and after decongestion to determine the difference between mucosal congestion and structural deformity.[6,20] AR also overestimates the cross-sectional area in locations farther than 5 cm from the nostrils, requires specialized equipment, experienced operators, and is sensitive to variations in techniques and testing conditions.[13,19,21]

### Imaging Studies

Imaging studies such as CT and MRI can be used to directly measure the area and volume of the nasal airway. AR has been validated against imaging, and these modalities strongly correlate.[13–18,22,23] CT can be used to objectively define anatomic factors, such as the angle of the internal nasal valve and the angulation and degree of septal deviation.[24] However, with respect to the latter, NOSE (nasal obstruction symptom evaluation) scores poorly correlated with CT findings, and there was poor concordance between side of obstructive symptoms reported by patients and the side of septal deviation on CT.[25]

Imaging limitations include that, like AR, they are static measurements and prone to changes in volume and area depending on the level of nasal congestion.[1,22,23] The nasal valve compromise clinical consensus recommends against the use of imaging in nasal obstruction diagnosis in favor of physical examination findings.[1] CT also can be used in nasal computational fluid dynamics, which are discussed later in this article.

### Clinician-Derived Outcomes

Clinician-derived outcome measures are based on quantifiable physical examination findings. These include direct visualization of nasal structures with anterior rhinoscopy, changes in obstructive symptoms with the Cottle or modified Cottle maneuver, and observation of the nasal wall during inspiration.[1] The Cottle maneuver, which involves widening the nasal valve by applying lateral pressure to the nasal sidewall or medial maxilla, has been found to have high sensitivity, but poor specificity in evaluating nasal obstruction.[26] However, the modified Cottle maneuver, which involves using a small item, such as an ear curette or cotton tip applicator to support the lateral nasal wall during inspiration, has been found to correlate significantly with airway improvement on placement of spreader grafts.[27] Nonetheless, physical examination findings are subjective and prone to bias. Although observer assessments are found to be sensitive for identifying anatomic deformities, they have low specificity in relation to subjective measures, meaning that clinicians may identify deformities that are not clinically significant.[28]

A grading system has been developed and validated for lateral wall insufficiency (LWI). These grades are based on 2 zones of the lateral nasal wall: zone 1 is defined as the lateral nasal wall superior to the scroll region of the upper and lower lateral cartilages, and zone 2 is defined as the lateral nasal wall inferior to the scroll area, primarily composing the ala (**Fig. 1**).[29,30] The grading system describes the degree of collapse on a scale of 0 to 3 (**Table 1**). In analyzing outcomes after surgical repair of LWI using both the validated LWI grading scale and NOSE scores, LWI scores and NOSE scores improved after functional rhinoplasty in both zones 1 and 2. There was also a positive linear correlation between LWI score and NOSE score, with the strongest between preoperative zone 1 and NOSE scores.[31] Moreover, a recent systematic review and meta-analysis of 10 studies evaluating the role of functional

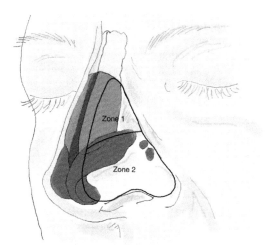

**Fig. 1.** Zones of LWI. LWI in zone 1 corresponds to lateral wall collapse above the scroll region, whereas zone 2 corresponds to lateral wall collapse below the scroll region.

| Table 1 | |
|---|---|
| **Lateral wall insufficiency grade** | |
| Grade | Degree of Collapse, % |
| 0 | No collapse |
| 1 | 1–33 |
| 2 | 34–66 |
| 3 | 67–100 |

*Data from* Tsao GJ, Fijalkowski N, Most SP. Validation of a grading system for lateral nasal wall insufficiency. Allergy Rhinol (Providence) 2013;4(2):e66–8.

rhinoplasty to treat LWI showed overall improvement of NOSE scores following surgery after pooled analysis.[32]

A validated grading system has similarly been developed for the size of the anterior inferior turbinates. This scale is graded from 1 to 4 based on the percentage of space occupied by the anterior inferior turbinate relative to the nasal cavity (**Table 2**).

## PHYSIOLOGIC OUTCOME MEASURES
### Rhinomanometry

Rhinomanometry measures transnasal pressure and nasal airflow to determine nasal airway resistance during inspiration.[33] Techniques include active and passive methods, as well as anterior and posterior methods. The active technique uses patients' own respiration for airflow, whereas the passive technique applies pressure to the nasal cavity via face mask.[34] The most commonly used technique is the more physiologic active anterior method.[19] During this method, the patient breathes through one nasal cavity and transnasal pressure, or the difference in pressure from the naris to the nasopharynx, is measured with a pressure transducer in the contralateral nostril.[6,34] Four-phase rhinomanometry, which gauges changes throughout the breathing cycle, is an emerging modality. It is reminiscent of pulmonary flow-volume loops, as it measures an accelerating inspiratory phase, decelerating inspiratory phase, accelerating expiratory phase, and decelerating expiratory phase. An advantage of this method is that it may yield additional diagnostic information regarding movement of the lateral wall and vestibule during breathing; however, it requires supraphysiologic pressures during forced respiration to obtain measurements.[19]

Advantage of anterior active rhinomanometry over the previously mentioned modalities include that it occurs during respiration and thus is dynamic, it measures nasal ventilation, and there is no distortion of the nasal vestibule, which can occur with AR.[19] Limitations of this techniques include the inability to precisely locate areas of

| Table 2 | |
|---|---|
| **Inferior turbinate grade** | |
| Grade | Percentage of Nasal Cavity Occupied by Inferior Turbinate |
| 1 | 0–25 |
| 2 | 26–50 |
| 3 | 51–75 |
| 4 | 76–100 |

*Data from* Camacho M, Zaghi S, Certal V, et al. Inferior turbinate classification system, grades 1 to 4: development and validation study. Laryngoscope 2015;125(2):296–302.

obstruction, its time-consuming nature, the need for specialized equipment and a well-trained operator, and that it cannot be performed in the presence of a septal perforation or if one nasal cavity is completely obstructed.[19,35] However, anterior active rhinomanometry is still considered the gold standard for objective assessments of the nasal airway.[19]

### Nasal Peak Inspiratory Flow

Nasal peak inspiratory flow (NPIF) measures the maximum airflow a patient is able to produce during forced nasal inspiration and is a measure of nasal patency.[36] It has been validated against rhinomanometry.[8,36] In relation to outcomes after rhinoplasty, NPIF has been shown to improve with the placement of spreader grafts.[37] Limitations of this technique include conflicting reproducibility and validity in structural and mucosal nasal disease. For example, it has been shown to miss approximately 25% of symptomatic patients with functionally relevant nasal structural deformity.[38] Additionally, confounding patient factors such as respiratory effort and pulmonary function status may adversely impact the results.[39]

### Computational Fluid Dynamics

Computational fluid dynamics (CFD) involves creating 3-dimensional computational models of patients' airways generated from imaging data such as CT or MRI. CFD software programs are then used to compute parameters such as nasal airflow, nasal resistance, heat transfer, and humidification. Advantages of this technique are that it can determine precise locations of nasal obstruction. Disadvantages include cost, and the specialization and time required to produce these models.[40–42] Studies have been performed to correlate data with other nasal obstruction subjective and objective measures, as well as for virtual surgery planning to predict surgical interventions that may have the most benefit for improving nasal obstruction.[40,43–45] Compared with acoustic rhinometry, its measurement of minimum cross-sectional area is more physiologic, as CFD finds the cross-section of airflow streams as opposed to AR, which finds the cross-sectional area perpendicular to the acoustic path.[45]

## PATIENT-REPORTED OUTCOME MEASURES

PROMs evaluate the subjective experience of the patient and the patient's self-reported assessment of the efficacy of a treatment without interpretation of the physician or others.[46] Thus, PROMs provide a quantitative assessment of otherwise subjective results. Those used for nasal obstruction are disease-specific, as nasal surgery outcomes may be too subtle for global quality-of-life (QOL) measures.[47] Both the nasal valve compromise and rhinoplasty clinical practice guidelines recommend the routine use of PROMs to gauge symptom severity and success of surgical intervention.[1,7,48] However, in a systematic review of rhinoplasty outcomes by Rhee and colleagues,[49] it was found that only 14% (6 total) of published functional rhinoplasty outcome studies involved the use of validated PROMs.[50] Despite this finding, the NOSE score is currently the most widely used validated PROM to evaluate functional rhinoplasty results.

In a recent systematic review of PROMs for rhinoplasty surgery, 10 surgery-specific questionnaires were identified: 3 functional rhinoplasty assessments, 3 aesthetic rhinoplasty assessments, and 4 combined functional and aesthetic assessments (**Table 3**). These include functional-only and combined functional-cosmetic measures, both of which are discussed in the following sections. The ideal PROM would be psychometrically validated and allow for comparison between interventions,

| Table 3 | |
|---|---|
| **Surgery-specific questionnaires for rhinoplasty assessment** | |
| **Type** | **Questionnaire** |
| Functional rhinoplasty only | Nasal Obstruction Symptoms Evaluation Scale (NOSE Scale) |
| | Nasal Obstruction Septoplasty Effectiveness (NOSE) |
| | Nasal Surgical Questionnaire (NSQ) |
| Aesthetic rhinoplasty only | Glasgow Benefit Inventory (GBI) |
| | FACE-Q Rhinoplasty Module (FACE-Q RM) |
| | Utrecht Questionnaire (UQ) |
| Combined functional and aesthetic rhinoplasty | Rhinoplasty Outcomes Evaluation (ROE) |
| | Functional Rhinoplasty Outcome Inventory 17 (FROI-17) |
| | Evaluation of Aesthetic Rhinoplasty Scale (EARS) |
| | Rhino Scale (RS) |

*Data from* Barone M, Cogliandro A, DiStefano N, et al. A systematic review of patient-reported outcome measures after rhinoplasty. Eur Arch Otorhinolaryngol 2017;274(4):1807–11.

quantification of positive effects, identification of patients most likely to benefit from a procedure, and provide follow-up standards and benchmarks for clinical studies.[51] The Standardized Cosmesis and Health Nasal Outcomes Survey (SCHNOS) was developed to provide a PROM that meets these criteria and is discussed further as follows.[3]

### Functional-Only PROMs

The NOSE score is a disease-specific QOL instrument developed for the assessment of nasal obstruction shown to be valid, reliable, and sensitive in evaluation of nasal obstruction.[4] The questionnaire has 5 questions based on a 4-point scale, with scores reported on a scale of 0 to 100 (raw score multiplied by 5) (**Fig. 2**). It was validated originally with patients undergoing septoplasty, and has been used in many subsequent studies of functional rhinoplasty as well.[4,36,47,52–56] A severity classification of the

**To the Patient:** Please help us to better understand the impact of nasal obstruction on your quality of life by <u>completing the following survey</u>. Thank you!

Over the past <u>ONE month</u>, how much of a <u>problem</u> were the following conditions for you?

Please circle the most correct response

| | Not a Problem | Very Mild Problem | Moderate Problem | Fairly Bad Problem | Severe Problem |
|---|---|---|---|---|---|
| 1. Nasal congestion or stuffiness | 0 | 1 | 2 | 3 | 4 |
| 2. Nasal blockage or obstruction | 0 | 1 | 2 | 3 | 4 |
| 3. Trouble breathing through my nose | 0 | 1 | 2 | 3 | 4 |
| 4. Trouble sleeping | 0 | 1 | 2 | 3 | 4 |
| 5. Unable to get enough air through my nose during exercise or exertion | 0 | 1 | 2 | 3 | 4 |

**Fig. 2.** NOSE scale. (*Adapted from* Stewart MG, Witsell DL, Smith TL, et al. Development and validation of the nasal obstruction symptom evaluation (NOSE) scale. Otolaryngol Head Neck Surg 2004;130:162; with permission.)

NOSE scale (mild: 5–25, moderate: 30–50, severe: 55–75, and extreme: >80), was developed and shown to have greater than 90% sensitivity and specificity in evaluation of patients with nasal airway obstruction.[56]

Another measure used is the nasal obstruction visual analog scale (VAS), which rates nasal obstruction on a continuous scale from 0 to 10 with the reported outcome as the closest integer.[36,57,58] Multiple studies show improvement in nasal obstruction VAS after surgical intervention, and one additional benefit of this scale is that it can be separated into left and right sided obstruction scales to evaluate unilateral symptoms as well.[49,59–62]

There are also several validated QOL measures focusing on inflammatory nasal disease such as the Rhinosinusitis Disability Index and SNOT-22.[63–65] As their primary goal is to evaluate inflammatory nasal disease, nasal obstructive measured by these instruments is more often secondary to inflammatory disease, rather than a structural abnormality. Additionally, despite concerns that functional rhinoplasty results are too subtle to impact global QOL measures, one recent study evaluating the EuroQOL5-dimension questionnaire did find clinically significant global health related QOL improvement following functional rhinoplasty.[66]

### Combined Functional and Cosmetic PROMs

Four combined functional and cosmetic PROMs were identified by systemic review, which include the Rhinoplasty Outcomes Evaluation (ROE), Functional Rhinoplasty Outcomes Inventory (FROI-17), RHINO scale, and Evaluation of Aesthetic Rhinoplasty Scale (EARS).[5,51,67–69] A recent study evaluating the impact of nasal obstruction on cosmetic results in patients undergoing combined functional and cosmetic rhinoplasty, compared the ROE and NOSE scores, as well as rhinomanometry. Interestingly, patients complaining of postoperative nasal obstruction and experienced both higher NOSE scores and increased resistance on rhinomanometry, and had worse aesthetic results compared with those without obstruction. Thus, nasal obstruction may have a significant impact on patients' aesthetic results as well.[70]

As stated previously, the SCHNOS was developed to address deficiencies in the previously discussed PROMs and to include both cosmetic and aesthetic rhinoplasty outcome measures.[3,51] The survey was extensively psychometrically and field-tested and includes 10 items rated on a Likert scale of 0 to 5.[3] Items included in this PROM can be seen in **Table 4**. This new tool is currently undergoing further validation and comparative studies to the previously discussed nasal obstruction measurement modalities.

## COMPARISON OF SUBJECTIVE AND OBJECTIVE OUTCOMES MEASURES

Despite many studies showing improvement of various nasal obstruction outcome measures following functional rhinoplasty procedures, controversy remains regarding the correlation between changes in objective and subjective outcome measures. Several studies have been published regarding this topic with variable results. Most investigations have not revealed any significant correlations.[61,62,71–80] For example, Lam and colleagues[36] compared AR, nasal peak inspiratory flow, nasal obstruction VAS, and the NOSE scale, and found no significant correlation between pooled objective and subjective measures, nor between anatomic (AR) or physiologic (NPIF) measures. Similarly, Andrews and colleagues[58] compared NPIF, SNOT-22, NOSE, and nasal obstruction VAS postoperatively. They found that although both objective and subjective outcome measures improved postoperatively, there was no significant correlation between them. However, Kjaergaard and colleagues[20] did find highly

**Table 4**
**Standardized cosmesis and health nasal outcomes survey (SCHNOS)**

*Over the past month, how much of a problem was the following:*

| | | No problem | | | | | Extreme problem |
|---|---|---|---|---|---|---|---|
| 1. | Having a blocked or obstructed nose | 0 | 1 | 2 | 3 | 4 | 5 |
| 2. | Getting air through my nose during exercise | 0 | 1 | 2 | 3 | 4 | 5 |
| 3. | Having a congested nose | 0 | 1 | 2 | 3 | 4 | 5 |
| 4. | Breathing through my nose during sleep | 0 | 1 | 2 | 3 | 4 | 5 |
| 5. | Decreased mood and self-esteem due to my nose | 0 | 1 | 2 | 3 | 4 | 5 |
| 6. | The shape of my nasal tip | 0 | 1 | 2 | 3 | 4 | 5 |
| 7. | The straightness of my nose | 0 | 1 | 2 | 3 | 4 | 5 |
| 8. | The shape of my nose from the side | 0 | 1 | 2 | 3 | 4 | 5 |
| 9. | How well my nose suits my face | 0 | 1 | 2 | 3 | 4 | 5 |
| 10. | The overall symmetry of my nose | 0 | 1 | 2 | 3 | 4 | 5 |

*From* Moubayed SP, Ioannidis JPA, Saltychev M, et al. The 10-item standardized cosmesis and health nasal outcomes survey (SCHNOS) for functional and cosmetic rhinoplasty. JAMA Facial Plast Surg 2018;20(1):39; with permission.

significant associations between subjective nasal obstruction VAS and objective AR and NPIF data. To further analyze this topic, a systematic review was conducted of 16 studies regarding the correlation of objective and subjective nasal obstruction outcome measures. Equivocal data were found, but data suggested that the chance of correlation is greater when each nasal passage is assessed individually, and when obstructive symptoms are present.[6]

There are several possible explanations for the lack of correlation between subjective and objective outcome measures. First, objective outcome measures are taken at one time point, whereas subjective outcome measures, such as the NOSE scale, ask patients to average symptoms over a period of 4 weeks. Thus, dynamic factors, such as nasal congestion or the nasal cycle, need to be taken into account.[36] To address the nasal cycle, a model using CFD simulating the midpoint of the nasal cycle was created and found to have increased correlation to nasal obstruction VAS and NOSE scores preoperatively and postoperatively compared with when this correction was not made.[44] Second, unilateral nasal obstruction may confound results, as one study found that if the difference in nasal resistance between 2 sides of the nose is less than 60% to 70%, it is difficult for patients to consistently detect the more obstructed side.[81] As shown by the systematic review, the correlation is improved when each side was individually assessed. It is important to remember, however, that most subjective measures, except the nasal obstruction VAS, do not differentiate between sides.[6] Although overall assessment of nasal obstruction is more clinically relevant, this may explain discordance between objective and subjective measurements. Finally, patients with symptomatic nasal obstruction also had greater correlation between objective and subjective measures, compared with asymptomatic patients.[6] Garcia and colleagues[45] performed an analysis using CFD to understand the relationship among nasal resistance, minimum cross-sectional area, and subjective measures, based on the theory that resistance only correlated with minimum cross-sectional area in severely constricted nasal cavities. They defined a minimum critical area of 0.37 $cm^2$. Areas smaller than this, which rarely occur in healthy individuals, are associated with nasal obstruction. Therefore, those with more symptomatic and severely constricted airways have greater chance of correlation between objective and subjective measures, whereas those with more subtle obstruction are less likely to show correlations between these measures.

## SUMMARY

Despite discordance between subjective and objective measures, the use of validated nasal obstruction outcome measures is essential in assessing the efficacy of interventions to treat obstruction. It is important to understand the different types of measurements available, as well as the advantages and limitations of each method to interpret their use in study results and assess one's own surgical outcomes. These validated measures provide the basis of evidence-based treatment of nasal airway obstruction and research.

## REFERENCES

1. Rhee JS, Weaver EM, Park SS, et al. Clinical consensus statement: diagnosis and management of nasal valve compromise. Otolaryngol Head Neck Surg 2010; 143(1):48–59.
2. Recker C, Hamilton GS. Evaluation of the patient with nasal obstruction. Facial Plast Surg 2016;32(1):3–8.
3. Moubayed SP, Ionnidis JPA, Saltychev M, et al. The 10-item standardized cosmesis and health nasal outcomes survey (SCHNOS) for functional and cosmetic rhinoplasty. JAMA Facial Plast Surg 2018;20(1):37–42.
4. Stewart MG, Witsell DL, Smith TL, et al. Development and validation of the nasal obstruction symptom evaluation (NOSE) scale. Otolaryngol Head Neck Surg 2004;130(2):157–63.
5. Lee MK, Most SP. A comprehensive quality-of-life instrument for aesthetic and functional rhinoplasty: the RHINO scale. Plast Reconstr Surg Glob Open 2016; 4(2):e611.
6. Andre RF, Vuyk HD, Ahmed A, et al. Correlation between subjective and objective evaluation of the nasal airway. A systematic review of the highest level of evidence. Clin Otolaryngol 2009;34(6):518–25.
7. Ishii LE, Tollefson TT, Basura GJ, et al. Clinical practice guideline: improving nasal form and function after rhinoplasty executive summary. Otolaryngol Head Neck Surg 2017;156(2):205–19.
8. Hilberg O. Objective measurement of nasal airway dimensions using acoustic rhinometry: methodological and clinical aspects. Allergy 2002;57(Suppl 70): 5–39.
9. Hilberg O, Pedersen OF. Acoustic rhinometry: recommendations for technical specifications and standard operating procedures. Rhinol Suppl 2000;16: 3–17.
10. Fisher EW, Morris DP, Biemans JM, et al. Practical aspects of acoustic rhinometry: problems and solutions. Rhinology 1995;33(4):219–33.

11. Parvez L, Erasala G, Noronha A. Novel techniques, standardization tools to enhance reliability of acoustic rhinometry measures. Rhinol Suppl 2000;16:18–28.

12. Wilson AM, Fowler SJ, Martin SW, et al. Evaluation of the importance of head and probe stabilisation in acoustic rhinometry. Rhinology 2001;39(2):93–7.

13. Terheyden H, Maune S, Mertens J, et al. Acoustic rhinometry: validation by three-dimensionally reconstructed computed tomographic scans. J Appl Physiol (1985) 2000;89(3):1013–21.

14. Hilberg O, Jensen FT, Pedersen OF. Nasal airway geometry: comparison between acoustic reflections and magnetic resonance scanning. J Appl Physiol (1985) 1993;75(6):2811–9.

15. Corey JP, Gungor A, Nelson R, et al. A comparison of the nasal cross-sectional areas and volumes obtained with acoustic rhinometry and magnetic resonance imaging. Otolaryngol Head Neck Surg 1997;117(4):349–54.

16. Corey JP, Nalbone VP, Ng BA. Anatomic correlates of acoustic rhinometry as measured by rigid nasal endoscopy. Otolaryngol Head Neck Surg 1999;121(5):572–6.

17. Min YG, Jan YJ. Measurements of cross-sectional area of the nasal cavity by acoustic rhinometry and CT scanning. Laryngoscope 1955;105:757–9.

18. Mamikoglu B, House S, Akbar I, et al. Acoustic rhinometry and computed tomography scans for diagnosis of nasal septal deviation, with clinical correlation. Otolaryngol Head Neck Surg 2000;123:61–8.

19. Clement PA, Halewyck S, Gordts F, et al. Critical evaluation of different objective techniques of nasal airway assessment: a clinical review. Eur Arch Otorhinolaryngol 2014;271(10):2617–25.

20. Kjaergaard T, Cvancarova M, Steinsvag SK. Does nasal obstruction mean that the nose is obstructed? Laryngoscope 2008;118(8):1476–81.

21. Clement PA, Gordts F. Standardisation committee on objective assessment of the nasal airway, IRS, ERS. Consensus report on acoustic rhinometry and rhinomanometry. Rhinology 2005;43(3):169–79.

22. Dastidar P, Numminen J, Heinonen T, et al. Nasal airway volumetric measurement using segmented HRCT images and acoustic rhinometry. Am J Rhinol 1999; 13(2):97–103.

23. Cakmak O, Coskun M, Celik H, et al. Value of acoustic rhinometry for measuring nasal valve area. Laryngoscope 2003;113(2):295–302.

24. Poetker DM, Rhee JS, Mocan BO, et al. Computed tomography technique for evaluation of nasal valve. Arch Facial Plast Surg 2004;6(4):240–3.

25. Ardeshirpour F, McCarn KE, McKinney AM, et al. Computed tomography scan does not correlate with patient experience of nasal obstruction. Laryngoscope 2016;126(4):820–5.

26. Tikanto J, Pirila T. Effects of the Cottle's maneuver on the nasal valve as assessed by acoustic rhinometry. Am J Rhinol 2007;21(4):456–9.

27. Fung E, Hong P, Moore C, et al. The effectiveness of modified Cottle maneuver in predicting outcomes in functional rhinoplasty. Plast Surg Int 2014;2014:618313.

28. Boyce JM, Eccles R. Assessment of subjective scales for selection of patients for nasal septal surgery. Clin Otolaryngol 2006;31(4):297–302.

29. Most SP. Trends in functional rhinoplasty. Arch Facial Plast Surg 2008;10(6):410–3.

30. Most SP. Comparing methods for repair of the external valve: one more step toward a unified view of lateral wall insufficiency. JAMA Facial Plast Surg 2015; 17(5):345–6.

31. Vaezeafshar R, Moubayed SP, Most SP. Repair of lateral wall insufficiency. JAMA Facial Plast Surg 2018;20(2):111–5.

32. Kandathil CK, Spataro EA, Laimi K, et al. Repair of the lateral nasal wall in nasal airway obstruction: a systematic review and meta-analysis. JAMA Facial Plast Surg 2018. https://doi.org/10.1001/jamafacial.2018.0036.

33. Naito K, Iwata S. Current advances in rhinomanometry. Eur Arch Otorhinolaryngol 1997;254(7):309–12.

34. Jones AS, Lancer JM, Stevens JC, et al. Rhinomanometry: do the anterior and posterior methods give equivalent results? Clin Otolaryngol Allied Sci 1987; 12(2):109–14.

35. Chandra RK, Patadia MO, Raviv J. Diagnosis of nasal airway obstruction. Otolaryngol Clin North Am 2009;42(2):207–25.

36. Lam DJ, James KT, Weaver EM. Comparison of anatomic, physiologic and subjective measures of the nasal airway. Am J Rhinol 2006;20(5):463–70.

37. Xavier R. Does rhinoplasty improve nasal breathing? Facial Plast Surg 2010; 26(4):328–32.

38. Bermuller C, Kirshce H, Rettinger G, et al. Diagnostic accuracy of peak nasal inspiratory flow and rhinomanometry in functional rhinosurgery. Laryngoscope 2008;118(4):605–10.

39. Angelos PC, Been MJ, Toriumi DM. Contemporary review of rhinoplasty. Arch Facial Plast Surg 2012;14(4):238–47.

40. Rhee JS, Pawar SS, Garcia GJ, et al. Toward personalized nasal surgery using computational fluid dynamics. Arch Facial Plast Surg 2011;13(5):305–10.

41. Pawar SS, Gacia GJ, Kimbell JS, et al. Objective measures in aesthetic and functional nasal surgery: perspectives on nasal form and function. Facial Plast Surg 2010;26(4):320–7.

42. Garcia GJ, Rhee JS, Senior BA. Septal deviation and nasal resistance: an investigation using virtual surgery and computational fluid dynamics. Am J Rhinol Allergy 2010;24(1):e46–53.

43. Casey KP, Borojeni AA, Koenig LJ, et al. Correlation between subjective nasal patency and intranasal airflow distribution. Otolaryngol Head Neck Surg 2017; 156(4):741–50.

44. Gaberino C, Rhee JS, Garcia GJ. Estimates of nasal airflow at the nasal cycle mid-point improve the correlation between objective and subjective measures of nasal patency. Respir Physiol Neuobiol 2017;238:23–32.

45. Garcia GJM, Hariri BM, Patel RG, et al. The relationship between nasal resistance to airflow and the airspace minimal cross-sectional area. J Biomech 2016;49(9):1670–8.

46. Lasch KE, Marquis P, Vigneux M, et al. PRO development: rigorous quantitative research as the crucial foundation. Qual Life Res 2010;19(8):1087–96.

47. Biggs TC, Fraser LR, Ward MJ, et al. Patient reported outcome measures in septorhinoplasty surgery. Ann R Coll Surg Engl 2015;97(1):63–5.

48. Most SP. The rhinoplasty clinical practice guideline: neither a cookbook for, recipe of, nor reduction sauce of the complex art of rhinoplasty. JAMA Facial Plast Surg 2017;19(2):85–6.

49. Rhee JS, Arganbright JM, McMullin BT, et al. Evidence supporting functional rhinoplasty or nasal valve repair: a 25 year systematic review. Otolaryngol Head Neck Surg 2008;139(1):10–20.

50. Floyd EM, Ho S, Patel P, et al. Systematic review and meta-analysis of studies evaluating functional rhinoplasty outcomes with the NOSE score. Otolaryngol Head Neck Surg 2017;156(6):809–15.

51. Barone M, Cogliandro A, DiStefano N, et al. A systematic review of patient-reported outcome measures after rhinoplasty. Eur Arch Otorhinolaryngol 2017; 274(4):1807–11.

52. Stewart MG, Smith TL, Weaver EM, et al. Outcomes after nasal septoplasty: results from the nasal obstruction septoplasty effectiveness (NOSE) study. Otolaryngol Head Neck Surg 2004;130(3):283–90.

53. Rhee JS, Poetker DM, Smith TL, et al. Nasal valve surgery improves disease-specific quality of life. Laryngoscope 2005;115(3):437–40.

54. Most SP. Analysis of outcomes after functional rhinoplasty using a disease-specific quality-of-life instrument. Arch Facial Plast Surg 2006;8(5):306–9.

55. Rhee JS, Sullivan CD, Frank DO, et al. A systematic review of patient-reported nasal obstruction scores: defining normative and symptomatic ranges in surgical patients. JAMA Facial Plast Surg 2014;16(3):219–25.

56. Lipan MJ, Most SP. Development of a severity classification system for subjective nasal obstruction. JAMA Facial Plast Surg 2013;15(5):358–61.

57. Cannon DE, Rhee JS. Evidence based practice: functional rhinoplasty. Otolaryngol Clin North Am 2012;45(5):1033–43.

58. Andrews PJ, Choudhury N, Takhar A, et al. The need for an objective measure in septorhinoplasty surgery: are we any closer to finding an answer? Clin Otolaryngol 2015;40(6):698–708.

59. Spielmann PM, White PS, Hussain SS. Surgical techniques for the treatment of nasal valve collapse: a systematic review. Laryngoscope 2009;119(7):1281–90.

60. Clarke JD, Hopkins ML, Eccles R. Evidence for correlation of objective and subjective measures of nasal airflow in patients with common cold. Clin Otolaryngol 2005;30(1):35–8.

61. Sipila J, Suonpaa J, Silvoniemi P, et al. Correlations between subjective sensation of nasal patency and rhinomanometry in both unilateral and total nasal assessment. ORL J Otorhinolaryngol Relat Spec 1995;57(5):260–3.

62. Hirschberg A, Rezek O. Correlation between objective and subjective assessments of nasal patency. ORL J Otorhinolaryngol Relat Spec 1998;60(4):206–11.

63. Benninger MS, Senior BA. The development of the rhinosinusitis disability index. Arch Otolaryngol Head Neck Surg 1997;123(11):1175–9.

64. Senior BA, Glaze C, Benninger MS. Use of the rhinosinusitis disability index (RSDI) in rhinologic disease. Am J Rhinol 2001;15(1):15–20.

65. Hopkins C, Gillett S, Slack R, et al. Psychometric validity of the 22-item sinonasal outcome test. Clin Otolaryngol 2009;34(5):447–54.

66. Fuller JC, Levesque PA, Lindsay RW. Assessment of the euroQol5-dimension questionnaire for detection of clinically significant global health-related quality-of-life improvement following functional septorhinoplasty. JAMA Facial Plast Surg 2017;19(2):95–100.

67. Alsarraf R. Outcomes research in facial plastic surgery: a review and new directions. Aesthetic Plast Surg 2000;24(3):192–7.

68. Balut C, Wallner F, Plinkert PK, et al. Development and validation of the functional rhinoplasty outcome inventory 17. Rhinology 2014;52(4):315–9.

69. Naraghi M, Atari M. Development and validation of the expectations of aesthetic rhinoplasty scale. Arch Plast Surg 2016;43(4):365–70.

70. Radulesco T, Penicaud M, Santini L, et al. Outcomes of septorhinoplasty: a new approach comparing functional and aesthetic results. Int J Oral Maxillofac Surg 2018;47(2):175–9.

71. Timperly D, Stow N, Srubiski A, et al. Functional outcomes of structured nasal tip refinement. Arch Facial Plast Surg 2010;12(5):298–304.

72. Fairley JW, Durham LH, Ell SR. Correlation of subjective sensation of nasal patency with nasal inspiratory peak flow rate. Clin Otolaryngol Allied Sci 1993; 18(1):19–22.

73. Wang DY, Raza MT, Goh DY, et al. Acoustic rhinometry in nasal allergen challenge study: which dimensional measures are meaningful? Clin Exp Allergy 2004;34(7):1093–8.
74. Larsen K, Kristensen S. Peak flow nasal patency indices and self-assessment in septoplasty. Clin Otolaryngol Allied Sci 1990;15(4):327–34.
75. Roithmann R, Cole P, Chapnik J, et al. Acoustic rhinometry, rhinomanometry, and the sensation of nasal patency: a correlative study. J Otolaryngol 1994;23(6):454–8.
76. Ozturk F, Turktas I, Asal K, et al. Effect of intranasal triamcinolone acetonide on bronchial hyper-responsiveness in children with seasonal allergic rhinitis and comparison of perceptional nasal obstruction with acoustic rhinometric assessment. Int J Pediatr Otorhinolaryngol 2004;68(8):1007–15.
77. Larsson C, Millqvist E, Bende M. Relationship between subjective nasal stuffiness and nasal patency measured by acoustic rhinometry. Am J Rhinol 2001;15(6):403–5.
78. Pirila T, Tikanto J. Unilateral and bilateral effects of nasal septum surgery demonstrated with acoustic rhinometry, rhinomanometry, and subjective assessment. Am J Rhinol 2001;15(2):127–33.
79. Jose J, Ell SR. The association of subjective nasal patency with peak inspiratory nasal flow in a large healthy population. Clin Otolaryngol Allied Sci 2003;28(4):352–4.
80. Rhee JS. Measuring outcomes in nasal surgery: realities and possibilities. Arch Facial Plast Surg 2009;11(6):416–9.
81. Sipila J, Suonpaa J, Laippala P. Sensation of nasal obstruction compared to rhinomanometric results in patients referred for septoplasty. Rhinology 1994;32(3):141–4.

# Medical Treatment of Nasal Airway Obstruction

Daniel R. Cox, MD, Sarah K. Wise, MD, MSCR*

## KEYWORDS

- Nasal obstruction • Medication • Pharmacotherapy • Intranasal corticosteroid
- Decongestant

## KEY POINTS

- Anatomic aberrations, structural deficiencies, nasal mucosal inflammation, and edema all contribute to nasal obstruction.
- Common causes of nasal mucosal inflammation include viral upper respiratory infections, allergic and nonallergic rhinitis, and nasal irritants.
- Medical therapy for nasal obstruction is aimed at controlling mucosal inflammation and swelling.
- Medications include topical and oral preparations. The choice of medical therapy depends on the underlying cause.

## OVERVIEW

Nasal airflow obstruction is often a multifactorial problem caused by a combination of anatomic aberrations, structural (bony/cartilaginous) weakness or deficiency, swelling of the nasal mucosa, and inferior turbinate enlargement. Anatomic and structural issues, such as nasal septal deviation and nasal valve collapse, are generally managed surgically. Medical therapy for nasal obstruction is directed at reducing nasal mucosal edema and inflammation.

Nasal obstruction occurs when swelling of the mucosa is sufficient to cause symptomatic blockage of airflow. Allergic rhinitis (AR), non-AR, and nasal polyposis are all examples of disease processes involving pathologic mucosal swelling and nasal obstruction that are improved with medical therapy.

Pharmacotherapy for nasal obstruction is aimed at reducing mucosal inflammation and/or edema. The medications used have various mechanisms of action and include systemic and topical preparations. This article discusses the most common medical

Disclosure Statement: None (D.R. Cox). Consultant for Elron, Medtronic, and OptiNose (S.K. Wise).
Department of Otolaryngology–Head and Neck Surgery, Emory University, 550 Peachtree Street, MOT 11th Floor, Atlanta, GA 30308, USA
* Corresponding author.
E-mail address: skmille@emory.edu

Otolaryngol Clin N Am 51 (2018) 897–908
https://doi.org/10.1016/j.otc.2018.05.004
0030-6665/18/© 2018 Elsevier Inc. All rights reserved.

therapies for nasal obstruction including current evidence on efficacy and side effect profile for each. This is summarized in **Table 1**.

## INTRANASAL CORTICOSTEROIDS

The most widely used medications in the management of nasal obstruction are the intranasal corticosteroids (INCS). The favorable safety and efficacy profile makes this class of medication an appropriate first-line selection for the most cases of nasal obstruction, regardless of the specific underlying cause. The mechanism through which corticosteroids decrease nasal inflammation is complex and incompletely understood. What is known is that they bind intracellular glucocorticoid receptors, resulting in upregulation of genes that encode anti-inflammatory mediators and cytokines and decreased transcription of proinflammatory genes.[1] They also inhibit recruitment of inflammatory cells to the nasal mucosa and decrease mucus production by goblet cells.

Numerous studies have been published that support the efficacy of INCS in the treatment of nasal airway obstruction. For example, one early study showed that after a 4-week course of therapy, intranasal budesonide reduced nasal airway resistance compared with placebo, as measured by subjective symptom scores and objective measures of nasal airway resistance.[2] A more recent randomized controlled trial (RCT) found that intranasal mometasone furoate significantly improved nasal obstruction symptom scores and peak nasal inspiratory flow compared with placebo after a 4-week course of treatment.[3] A 2008 meta-analysis of 16 RCTs comparing mometasone furoate with placebo found mometasone furoate to be superior.[4]

There are several different INCS agents currently available in the United States. Current evidence shows little difference in efficacy among the various INCS agents when used to treat seasonal AR (SAR).[5] For patients with perennial AR (PAR), there is some evidence that high-dose (256 μg every day) budesonide aqueous nasal spray may be more effective at relieving nasal obstruction than intranasal fluticasone propionate or mometasone furoate.[6] Budesonide nasal spray is also noted to be more cost effective than other agents.[7] In addition to nasal spray preparations, budesonide is frequently added to saline and delivered to the nasal mucosa via irrigation, particularly in patients with nasal polyps. There is evidence that this delivery method has a good safety and efficacy profile.[8,9]

Another important consideration that differentiates INCS sprays is patient preference related to the sensory experience associated with using these medications (ie, smell, taste, spray force). Results of patient preference studies suggest that budesonide and triamcinolone nasal sprays are preferred over fluticasone and mometasone sprays.[7]

Generally, an extended course of therapy (2–4 weeks) is recommended to reach full effect. There is, however, some evidence that INCS may demonstrate efficacy when used on an as-needed basis. In one RCT, patients with nasal polyposis receiving mometasone furoate nasal spray experienced a statistically significant improvement in peak nasal inspiratory flow by Day 2 of therapy and statistically significant symptomatic relief of nasal congestion by Day 3.[10]

The most common side effects of INCS include nasal irritation and discomfort, dryness, and epistaxis. Septal perforations have been associated with INCS use.[11] Concerns have been raised about the possibility of more serious side effects, such mucosal atrophy, glaucoma, cataracts, and hypothalamic-pituitary-adrenal (HPA) axis suppression; however, current evidence suggests that INCS use does not increase the risk of development of any of these complications. One study showed no evidence of HPA axis suppression with budesonide irrigation use out to 2 years

**Table 1**
Summary of medical therapies for nasal obstruction

| Drug Class | Common Agents | Mechanism | Common Side Effects | Major Side Effects | Relative Efficacy |
|---|---|---|---|---|---|
| INCS | Fluticasone propionate, mometasone furoate, budesonide aqueous, triamcinolone aqueous | Upregulation of anti-inflammatory genes and downregulation of proinflammatory genes in local tissues | Nasal irritation and discomfort, dryness, and epistaxis | Septal perforation, growth suppression (pediatric patients) | Preferred first-line therapy for most cases |
| Oral corticosteroids | Prednisone, dexamethasone, prednisolone, methylprednisolone | Systemic upregulation of anti-inflammatory genes and downregulation of proinflammatory genes | Weight gain, irritability, hyperglycemia | HPA axis suppression, cataracts, growth retardation, avascular hip necrosis | Roughly equivalent to INCS with less favorable side effect profile |
| INCI | Triamcinolone | Upregulation of anti-inflammatory genes and downregulation of proinflammatory genes in local tissues | Injection site bleeding, cheek flushing | Orbital complications including retinal embolization and blindness | Little data on head-to-head comparisons with other agents. Seems to be less effective than INB based on one study |
| OH1A | First generation: diphenhydramine, chlorpheniramine. Second generation: loratadine, cetirizine, desloratadine, levocetirizine | H1 histamine receptor blockade | Drowsiness, mucosal drying, headache, abdominal pain | Bronchospasm, hepatotoxicity, seizures, hemolytic anemia | Less effective than INCS, comparable efficacy with INA |
| Oral H2 antihistamines | Ranitidine, famotidine, cimetidine | H2 histamine receptor blockade | Headache, dry mouth | Thrombocytopenia, hepatotoxicity, pneumonia | Less effective than OH1A but may be an effective adjunctive therapy |
| INA | Azelastine, olopatadine | H1 histamine receptor blockade | Bitter taste, headache, drowsiness | Septal perforation, hyposmia/anosmia, depression | Comparable with INCS in patients with AR |

(continued on next page)

**Table 1**
*(continued)*

| Drug Class | Common Agents | Mechanism | Common Side Effects | Major Side Effects | Relative Efficacy |
|---|---|---|---|---|---|
| Oral decongestants | Pseudoephedrine, phenylephrine | Stimulation of α-adrenergic receptors resulting in vasoconstriction | Palpitations, tachycardia, urinary retention, anxiety, insomnia | Hypertension, arrythmias | Effective for acute episodes but long-term use is limited by side effects May be more effective in combination with OH1A |
| Topical decongestants | Oxymetazoline, phenylephrine | Stimulation of α-adrenergic receptors resulting in vasoconstriction | Nasal irritation, dryness, tachycardia, palpitations, restlessness | Rhinitis medicamentosa, arrhythmias, angina | Very effective for nasal obstruction but use is limited by concern for rebound |
| Intranasal botulinum toxin | Botulinum toxin A | Inhibits acetylcholine release from presynaptic nerve terminals | Headache, nasal dryness, epistaxis from injection site | Anaphylaxis, effect spread: asthenia, weakness, blurred vision, diplopia | Superior to INCI based on one study |
| Nasal saline | N/A | Cleanses nose, clears irritants and allergens | Nasal irritation | None | Less effective than INCS; however, excellent safety and tolerability profile makes this a first-line treatment option |
| Oral antileukotrienes | Montelukast, zafirlukast | Blockade of leukotriene receptors | Headache, flulike symptoms, fever, abdominal pain, cough, nausea, dyspepsia, anxiety, restlessness | Anaphylaxis, hepatic eosinophilic infiltration, Churg-Strauss, thrombocytopenia, neuropsychiatric disorders, pulmonary eosinophilia | Equivalent or slightly inferior to OH1A for nasal obstruction Generally used as a second- or third-line agent |

*Abbreviations:* HPA, hypothalamic-pituitary-adrenal axis; INA, intranasal antihistamines; INB, intranasal botulinum toxin A; INCI, intranasal steroid injection; INCS, intranasal corticosteroids; OH1A, oral H1 antihistamines.

duration of therapy.[9] There is some evidence that INCS may adversely affect growth velocity in children in the short term, but long-term effects are unclear.[12]

## ORAL CORTICOSTEROIDS

Oral corticosteroids are effective in the treatment of nasal obstruction, particularly in patients with nasal polyposis.[13] Because of the undesirable side effect profile of oral corticosteroids, topical preparations are generally preferred for management of nasal obstruction, except in cases where mucosal edema is expected to be short lived (ie, acute upper respiratory infection, perioperative period), or where obstruction is severe enough that penetration by topical agents is unlikely (ie, severe polyposis).[14,15]

Oral corticosteroids do not seem to offer any additional benefit in terms of efficacy compared with INCS in patients with AR. In a recent RCT of patients with SAR, loratadine plus intranasal mometasone furoate was equally effective as loratadine plus oral betamethasone at improving nasal symptoms.[16]

Known side effects of oral steroids include HPA axis suppression, cataracts, growth retardation, weight gain, irritability, avascular necrosis of the hip, and hyperglycemia, among others. These effects seem to be dose-dependent and are increasingly likely with long-term use. However, these reactions can be idiosyncratic and occur with minimal use. These agents should therefore be used judiciously and limited to short courses where possible.

## INTRANASAL STEROID INJECTIONS

Some early studies from the 1970s established the effectiveness of intranasal corticosteroid injection (INCI) in the treatment of nasal obstruction.[17,18] A more recent study published in the past 10 years showed that in patients with AR, injection with triamcinolone decreased nasal obstruction versus placebo.[19]

This treatment has fallen out of favor in recent years, because INCI has been associated with an increased risk of orbital complications. The mechanism of eye injury following INCI is not entirely clear. In at least one case, vision loss was associated with choroidal and retinal artery embolization believed to be via retrograde flow from the turbinate to the ophthalmic artery.[20] Related to this concern, a recent review found a low estimated visual complication rate of 0.003%.[21]

## ORAL H1 ANTIHISTAMINES

Histamine is an inflammatory mediator present in nasal mast cells that is released on allergen exposure. It exerts its effect on the nasal mucosa through interaction with histamine-specific receptors in nasal tissues. Four histamine receptor subtypes have been identified, H1 and H2 being the longest studied.[22]

H1 receptor stimulation is responsible for much of the symptomatology of AR including sneezing, itching, and rhinorrhea, and it is also believed to play a significant role in the pathophysiology of nasal obstruction in AR. H1 receptors are present on the endothelium of blood vessels in the inferior turbinate,[23] and H1 receptors have been shown to mediate vasodilation in human nasal blood vessels in vitro.[24]

It was traditionally believed that H1 antihistamines were ineffective in the treatment of nasal obstruction in AR. However, Hore and colleagues[25] found H1 antihistamines to be more effective than placebo at improving patient and health care worker assessed nasal obstruction scores. More recently, however, second-generation H1 antihistamines have been shown to be consistently effective at relieving nasal obstruction compared with placebo.[26]

H1 antihistamines are broadly classified into first- and second-generation agents. First-generation antihistamines, such as diphenhydramine and chlorpheniramine, are lipophilic and readily cross the blood-brain barrier, leading to central nervous system side effects including drowsiness, fatigue, impaired concentration, and memory problems. They also inhibit CYPD6 in the liver, resulting in impaired metabolism of some other medications. Second-generation H1 blockers, such as loratadine, cetirizine, and desloratadine, are more lipophobic, thus minimizing penetration of the blood-brain barrier and avoiding some of the common side effects associated with first-generation agents. Second-generation agents are generally well tolerated. Common side effects include headache, nausea, fatigue, nasal dryness, and dry mouth. Nonetheless, second-generation agents are typically preferred in most patients.

With respect to the efficacy of second-generation agents, a recent systematic review found that desloratadine, fexofenadine, and levocetirizine were significantly better than placebo at improving objective and subjective measures of nasal congestion.[26] Another recent systematic review showed that levocetirizine was consistently effective at treating nasal obstruction in AR, with the onset as early as 2 hours and lasting over 6 weeks.[27]

## ORAL H2 ANTIHISTAMINES

There is some evidence that H2 histamine receptor blockade is useful for treatment of AR with persistent nasal airway obstruction, even in those already being treated with oral H1 antihistamines. However, these data are limited and conflicting. One early RCT showed that patients pretreated with ranitidine experienced a smaller increase in nasal airway resistance after a histamine challenge compared with those pretreated with cetirizine[28] Taylor-Clark and coworkers[29] found that pretreatment with a combination of ranitidine and cetirizine caused greater inhibition of nasal blockage after histamine challenge than pretreatment with cetirizine alone. However, other studies failed to show an improvement in nasal obstruction with the addition of cimetidine.[30] Addition of oral H2 antihistamine to a patient treatment plan is at the treating physicians discretion.

## INTRANASAL ANTIHISTAMINES

Intranasal antihistamines have a distinct advantage over oral antihistamines; they avoid systemic side effects.[31] Azelastine and olopatadine are the two agents currently available in the United States.

Intranasal antihistamines are effective in the treatment of nasal obstruction, particularly in patients with AR as the underlying cause. In a recent study by Kalpaklioglu and Kavut,[32] azelastine, 0.56 mg twice a day, was comparable with triamcinolone acetonide spray at improving nasal peak inspiratory flow rate. Gastpar and colleagues[33] showed azelastine to be at least as effective as budesonide nasal spray at improving nasal symptoms; nasal flow rate was improved with both medications. There is emerging evidence that intranasal antihistamines are also efficacious for non-AR.[34]

Intranasal antihistamines are generally well tolerated and have a good side-effect profile. The most commonly reported side effect is the unpleasant taste. Epistaxis, headache, and nasal discomfort have also been reported.

## ORAL DECONGESTANTS

Oral decongestants are agents commonly found in over-the-counter cold remedies. They exert their decongestant effect on the nasal mucosa through $\alpha$-adrenergic stimulation resulting in vasoconstriction.

Available evidence suggests that oral decongestants are effective in the treatment of nasal obstruction. In one RCT, daily dosing of 240 mg of pseudoephedrine for 2 weeks resulted in significant improvement of nasal congestion from baseline.[35] In another RCT, patients suffering from an acute upper respiratory tract infection experienced significant improvement in objective and subjective measures of nasal obstruction after a single 60-mg dose of pseudoephedrine.[36]

The two main agents available in the United States are pseudoephedrine and phenylephrine. Studies comparing the two medications have demonstrated pseudoephedrine to be more effective. One RCT showed that pseudoephedrine was more effective than phenylephrine at relieving nasal obstruction, and that phenylephrine was not significantly better than placebo.[37] Meltzer and coworkers[38] also found that phenylephrine was no better than placebo at decreasing nasal congestion.

Studies have demonstrated significant blood pressure and/or heart rate increases with oral decongestant use, and these changes are more pronounced with immediate-release preparations.[39,40] Patients with underlying cardiovascular or cerebrovascular conditions should therefore be closely monitored when taking oral decongestants. Other common side effects include anxiety, insomnia, and tremors. In addition, oral decongestants have been linked to voiding dysfunction in male patients greater than 50 years of age.[41]

## TOPICAL DECONGESTANTS

Topical nasal decongestants act directly on $\alpha$-adrenergic receptors in the nasal mucosa to effect vasoconstriction and shrinkage of the nasal mucosa. Oxymetazoline and xylometazoline are the most common agents available in the United States.

Application of a topical nasal decongestant results in rapid, and often marked, improvement in nasal patency and airflow in patients with turbinate enlargement or mucosal edema. A recent RCT showed that xylometazoline was more effective at nasal decongestion than mometasone furoate as measured by objective and subjective measures.[42]

Although topical decongestants are extremely effective in the short term, their long-term usefulness is limited by the concern for development of rebound congestion with extended use, a condition known as rhinitis medicamentosa. This is a difficult condition to manage once it develops, so every effort should be made to avoid this problem. There is some debate in the literature regarding the duration of therapy required for rebound congestion to develop. Watanabe and colleagues[43] showed no evidence of rebound or loss of effect after a 4-week course. Conversely, in an RCT by Morris and colleagues,[44] rebound congestion was seen at 3 days after treatment initiation. Some authors have suggested that concomitant use of nasal steroid spray can reduce rebound congestion.[45]

## INTRANASAL BOTULINUM TOXIN INJECTIONS

Botulinum toxin A is an exotoxin produced by the bacterium *Clostridium botulinum*.[46] Its mechanism of action involves blocking acetylcholine release in presynaptic nerve terminals. It is used in the management of several neuromuscular disorders. Recent reports have been published on the use of intranasal botulinum toxin A (INB) injections for the treatment of AR and vasomotor rhinitis. An early study showed that INB was effective at relieving rhinorrhea in patients with vasomotor rhinitis but was not effective at relieving nasal obstruction.[47] Subsequent reports suggest that INB may be a viable option for managing nasal obstruction. In a recent RCT, Unal and colleagues[48] demonstrated that a single INB injection resulted in significant improvement in nasal obstruction compared with placebo, and this effect was sustained for up to 8 weeks after the injection. Another study compared INB injection with INCI, and found INB injection to be superior to INCI and placebo.[19]

There is some variability in the literature regarding injection location. Some authors describe inferior turbinate injection,[19] whereas others recommend both inferior and middle turbinate injection,[49] and still others have reported on injection of the posterior lateral nasal wall.[50] The recommended dose of toxin ranges from 10 to 20 units per side. One study showed no significant change when the dose was increased from 20 to 30 units.[48]

INB was well tolerated in the published studies. Common side effects included mild headache, mild nose dryness, and epistaxis.

## NASAL SALINE

Nasal saline comes in a variety of different compositions and concentrations including isotonic and hypertonic solutions, seawater, and buffered versus nonbuffered solutions. Nasal saline cleanses the nose, clearing irritants and allergens from the mucosal surface. In addition, some preparations have specific ingredients that may provide additional benefit. For example, it has been proposed that the magnesium in Dead Sea saline may have anti-inflammatory properties.[51] There are several delivery systems available and doses range from small-volume spray applications to large-volume (240–500 mL) irrigations.

Nasal saline is a particularly attractive treatment option for nasal obstruction because it is nonpharmacologic and has minimal side effects. In addition, there is evidence supporting the efficacy of nasal saline. Cordray and colleagues[51] demonstrated that in patients with SAR, use of Dead Sea spray resulted in significant improvement in all subdomains of the rhinoconjunctivitis quality of life questionnaire. Likewise, in an RCT of pregnant women with SAR, nasal resistance was significantly reduced at 3 and 6 weeks after initiation of hypertonic saline irrigation therapy.[52]

Common side effects include epistaxis, nasal discomfort, ear pain, and headache. Concerns have been raised about sinonasal infections secondary to contaminated saline irrigation delivery systems. In multiple studies, pathogenic organisms have been isolated from saline irrigation bottles; however, the clinical significance is unclear.[53] There is some evidence that disinfection procedures, such as cleaning with Milton solution or microwaving the delivery system, may reduce contamination.[54]

## ORAL ANTILEUKOTRIENES

Leukotrienes are a product of the 5-lipoxygenase metabolism of arachidonic acid, which occurs in leukocytes in response to antigen exposure in AR. Leukotrienes bind receptors on target cells, resulting in increased mucus secretion, congestion, and inflammation.[55] Leukotriene receptor antagonists (LTRAs), such as montelukast, block these receptors, decreasing nasal inflammation.

In an RCT of patients with PAR, Jiang[56] found that zafirlukast was superior to loratadine and a combination of loratadine and pseudoephedrine at reducing nasal obstruction scores. Mucha and colleagues[35] showed that montelukast was equivalent to pseudoephedrine at improving nasal peak inspiratory flow in patients with SAR. However, pseudoephedrine was superior to montelukast at improving the symptom of nasal congestion. In a recent systematic review, LTRAs were found to be superior to placebo but inferior to INCS at reducing nasal congestion in patients with SAR.[57] Similar results have been seen in patients with PAR.[58] Overall, LTRAs seem to be equivalent or slightly inferior to oral antihistamines in terms of efficacy.[57,58] They are also more expensive than oral antihistamines.[59]

LTRAs have a good safety profile and are generally well tolerated. Common side effects include headache, insomnia, cough, dry mouth, anxiety, heartburn, restlessness, and throat irritation.

## COMBINATION THERAPIES

For many patients with nasal obstruction amenable to medical management, monotherapy with a single agent is sufficient to adequately control symptoms. For patients with more recalcitrant symptoms, however, a combination of agents may be required. Some of the medication classes described in this article seem to work well in combination.

For example, there is some evidence that oral decongestants may be more effective when combined with oral H1 antihistamines. In a recent RCT, the combination of pseudoephedrine and cetirizine was found to be more effective than either agent alone.[60] Zieglmayer and colleagues[61] found that the combination of cetirizine and prolonged-release pseudoephedrine was more effective than budesonide nasal spray at relieving nasal obstruction during allergen exposure. Similarly, the combination of INCS and intranasal antihistamines seems to be more effective than placebo or either therapy alone in patients with AR.[62]

## SUMMARY

Medical management of nasal obstruction is aimed at reducing nasal mucosal inflammation and edema, thereby opening nasal passages and improving airflow. There are several different medication options to choose from and they can be used alone or in combination. Selection of an appropriate regimen depends on the underlying cause and patient preference factors.

## REFERENCES

1. Okano M. Mechanisms and clinical implications of glucocorticosteroids in the treatment of allergic rhinitis. Clin Exp Immunol 2009;158:164–73.
2. Henriksen JM, Wenzel A. Effect of an intranasally administered corticosteroid (budesonide) on nasal obstruction, mouth breathing, and asthma. Am Rev Respir Dis 1984;130:1014–8.
3. Meltzer EO, Munafo DA, Chung W, et al. Intranasal mometasone furoate therapy for allergic rhinitis symptoms and rhinitis-disturbed sleep. Ann Allergy Asthma Immunol 2010;105:65–74.
4. Penagos M, Compalati E, Tarantini F, et al. Efficacy of mometasone furoate nasal spray in the treatment of allergic rhinitis. Meta-analysis of randomized, double-blind, placebo-controlled, clinical trials. Allergy 2008;63:1280–91.
5. Gross G, Jacobs RL, Woodworth TH, et al. Comparative efficacy, safety, and effect on quality of life of triamcinolone acetonide and fluticasone propionate aqueous nasal sprays in patients with fall seasonal allergic rhinitis. Ann Allergy Asthma Immunol 2002;89:56–62.
6. Bende M, Carrillo T, Vona I, et al. A randomized comparison of the effects of budesonide and mometasone furoate aqueous nasal sprays on nasal peak flow rate and symptoms in perennial allergic rhinitis. Ann Allergy Asthma Immunol 2002; 88:617–23.

7. Herman H. Once-daily administration of intranasal corticosteroids for allergic rhinitis: a comparative review of efficacy, safety, patient preference, and cost. Am J Rhinol 2007;21:70–9.

8. Nader ME, Abou-Jaoude P, Cabaluna M, et al. Using response to a standardized treatment to identify phenotypes for genetic studies of chronic rhinosinusitis. J Otolaryngol Head Neck Surg 2010;39:69–75.

9. Smith KA, French G, Mechor B, et al. Safety of long-term high-volume sinonasal budesonide irrigations for chronic rhinosinusitis. Int Forum Allergy Rhinol 2016;6: 228–32.

10. Small CB, Stryszak P, Danzig M, et al. Onset of symptomatic effect of mometasone furoate nasal spray in the treatment of nasal polyposis. J Allergy Clin Immunol 2008;121:928–32.

11. Lanier B, Kai G, Marple B, et al. Pathophysiology and progression of nasal septal perforation. Ann Allergy Asthma Immunol 2007;99:473–9 [quiz: 480–1, 521].

12. Mener DJ, Shargorodsky J, Varadhan R, et al. Topical intranasal corticosteroids and growth velocity in children: a meta-analysis. Int Forum Allergy Rhinol 2015; 5:95–103.

13. Poetker DM, Jakubowski LA, Lal D, et al. Oral corticosteroids in the management of adult chronic rhinosinusitis with and without nasal polyps: an evidence-based review with recommendations. Int Forum Allergy rhinology 2013;3:104–20.

14. Bensch GW. Safety of intranasal corticosteroids. Ann Allergy Asthma Immunol 2016;117:601–5.

15. Jang TY, Kim YH. Recent updates on the systemic and local safety of intranasal steroids. Curr Drug Metab 2016;17:992–6.

16. Karaki M, Akiyama K, Mori N. Efficacy of intranasal steroid spray (mometasone furoate) on treatment of patients with seasonal allergic rhinitis: comparison with oral corticosteroids. Auris Nasus Larynx 2013;40:277–81.

17. Baker DC. Treatment of obstructing inferior turbinates with intranasal corticosteroids. Ann Plast Surg 1979;3:253–9.

18. Mabry RL. Intraturbinal steroid injection: indications, results, and complications. South Med J 1978;71:789–91, 794.

19. Yang TY, Jung YG, Kim YH, et al. A comparison of the effects of botulinum toxin A and steroid injection on nasal allergy. Otolaryngol Head Neck Surg 2008;139: 367–71.

20. Martin PA, Church CA, Petti GH Jr, et al. Visual loss after intraturbinate steroid injection. Otolaryngol Head Neck Surg 2003;128:280–1.

21. Moss WJ, Kjos KB, Karnezis TT, et al. Intranasal steroid injections and blindness: our personal experience and a review of the past 60 years. Laryngoscope 2015; 125:796–800.

22. Xie H, He SH. Roles of histamine and its receptors in allergic and inflammatory bowel diseases. World J Gastroenterol 2005;11:2851–7.

23. Nakaya M, Takeuchi N, Kondo K. Immunohistochemical localization of histamine receptor subtypes in human inferior turbinates. Ann Otol Rhinol Laryngol 2004; 113:552–7.

24. Birchall MA, Schroter RC, Pride NB. Changes in nasal mucosal blood flux and airflow resistance on unilateral histamine challenge. Clin Otolaryngol Allied Sci 1993;18:139–44.

25. Hore I, Georgalas C, Scadding G. Oral antihistamines for the symptom of nasal obstruction in persistent allergic rhinitis: a systematic review of randomized controlled trials. Clin Exp Allergy 2005;35:207–12.

26. Bachert C. A review of the efficacy of desloratadine, fexofenadine, and levocetirizine in the treatment of nasal congestion in patients with allergic rhinitis. Clin Ther 2009;31:921–44.

27. Patou J, De Smedt H, van Cauwenberge P, et al. Pathophysiology of nasal obstruction and meta-analysis of early and late effects of levocetirizine. Clin Exp Allergy 2006;36:972–81.

28. Wood-Baker R, Lau L, Howarth PH. Histamine and the nasal vasculature: the influence of H1 and H2-histamine receptor antagonism. Clin Otolaryngol Allied Sci 1996;21:348–52.

29. Taylor-Clark T, Sodha R, Warner B, et al. Histamine receptors that influence blockage of the normal human nasal airway. Br J Pharmacol 2005;144:867–74.

30. Juliusson S, Bende M. Effect of systemically administered H1- and H2-receptor antagonists on nasal blood flow as measured with laser Doppler flowmetry in a provoked allergic reaction. Rhinology 1996;34:24–7.

31. Davies RJ, Bagnall AC, McCabe RN, et al. Antihistamines: topical vs oral administration. Clin Exp Allergy 1996;26(Suppl 3):11–7.

32. Kalpaklioglu AF, Kavut AB. Comparison of azelastine versus triamcinolone nasal spray in allergic and nonallergic rhinitis. Am J Rhinol Allergy 2010;24:29–33.

33. Gastpar H, Aurich R, Petzold U, et al. Intranasal treatment of perennial allergic rhinitis. Comparison of azelastine nasal spray and budesonide nasal aerosol. Arzneimittelforschung 1993;43:475–9.

34. Daramola OO, Kern RC. An update regarding the treatment of nonallergic rhinitis. Curr Opin Otolaryngol Head Neck Surg 2016;24:10–4.

35. Mucha SM, deTineo M, Naclerio RM, et al. Comparison of montelukast and pseudoephedrine in the treatment of allergic rhinitis. Arch Otolaryngol Head Neck Surg 2006;132:164–72.

36. Eccles R, Jawad MS, Jawad SS, et al. Efficacy and safety of single and multiple doses of pseudoephedrine in the treatment of nasal congestion associated with common cold. Am J Rhinol 2005;19:25–31.

37. Horak F, Zieglmayer P, Zieglmayer R, et al. A placebo-controlled study of the nasal decongestant effect of phenylephrine and pseudoephedrine in the Vienna Challenge Chamber. Ann Allergy Asthma Immunol 2009;102:116–20.

38. Meltzer EO, Ratner PH, McGraw T. Oral phenylephrine HCl for nasal congestion in seasonal allergic rhinitis: a randomized, open-label, placebo-controlled study. J Allergy Clin Immunol Pract 2015;3:702–8.

39. Salerno SM, Jackson JL, Berbano EP. The impact of oral phenylpropanolamine on blood pressure: a meta-analysis and review of the literature. J Hum Hypertens 2005;19:643–52.

40. Salerno SM, Jackson JL, Berbano EP. Effect of oral pseudoephedrine on blood pressure and heart rate: a meta-analysis. Arch Intern Med 2005;165:1686–94.

41. Shao IH, Wu CC, Tseng HJ, et al. Voiding dysfunction in patients with nasal congestion treated with pseudoephedrine: a prospective study. Drug Des Devel Ther 2016;10:2333–9.

42. Barnes ML, Biallosterski BT, Gray RD, et al. Decongestant effects of nasal xylometazoline and mometasone furoate in persistent allergic rhinitis. Rhinology 2005;43:291–5.

43. Watanabe H, Foo TH, Djazaeri B, et al. Oxymetazoline nasal spray three times daily for four weeks in normal subjects is not associated with rebound congestion or tachyphylaxis. Rhinology 2003;41:167–74.

44. Morris S, Eccles R, Martez SJ, et al. An evaluation of nasal response following different treatment regimens of oxymetazoline with reference to rebound congestion. Am J Rhinol 1997;11:109–15.

45. Ferguson BJ, Paramaesvaran S, Rubinstein E. A study of the effect of nasal steroid sprays in perennial allergic rhinitis patients with rhinitis medicamentosa. Otolaryngol Head Neck Surg 2001;125:253–60.

46. Ozcan C, Ismi O. Botulinum toxin for rhinitis. Curr Allergy Asthma Rep 2016;16:58.

47. Kim KS, Kim SS, Yoon JH, et al. The effect of botulinum toxin type A injection for intrinsic rhinitis. J Laryngol Otol 1998;112:248–51.

48. Unal M, Sevim S, Dogu O, et al. Effect of botulinum toxin type A on nasal symptoms in patients with allergic rhinitis: a double-blind, placebo-controlled clinical trial. Acta Otolaryngol 2003;123:1060–3.

49. Ozcan C, Vayisoglu Y, Dogu O, et al. The effect of intranasal injection of botulinum toxin A on the symptoms of vasomotor rhinitis. Am J Otolaryngol 2006;27:314–8.

50. Zhang EZ, Tan S, Loh I. Botulinum toxin in rhinitis: literature review and posterior nasal injection in allergic rhinitis. Laryngoscope 2017;127:2447–54.

51. Cordray S, Harjo JB, Miner L. Comparison of intranasal hypertonic dead sea saline spray and intranasal aqueous triamcinolone spray in seasonal allergic rhinitis. Ear Nose Throat J 2005;84:426–30.

52. Garavello W, Somigliana E, Acaia B, et al. Nasal lavage in pregnant women with seasonal allergic rhinitis: a randomized study. Int Arch Allergy Immunol 2010;151:137–41.

53. Psaltis AJ, Foreman A, Wormald PJ, et al. Contamination of sinus irrigation devices: a review of the evidence and clinical relevance. Am J Rhinol Allergy 2012;26:201–3.

54. Keen M, Foreman A, Wormald PJ. The clinical significance of nasal irrigation bottle contamination. Laryngoscope 2010;120:2110–4.

55. Peters-Golden M, Henderson WR Jr. The role of leukotrienes in allergic rhinitis. Ann Allergy Asthma Immunol 2005;94:609–18 [quiz: 618–20, 669].

56. Jiang RS. Efficacy of a leukotriene receptor antagonist in the treatment of perennial allergic rhinitis. J Otolaryngol 2006;35:117–21.

57. Rodrigo GJ, Yanez A. The role of antileukotriene therapy in seasonal allergic rhinitis: a systematic review of randomized trials. Ann Allergy Asthma Immunol 2006;96:779–86.

58. Grainger J, Drake-Lee A. Montelukast in allergic rhinitis: a systematic review and meta-analysis. Clin Otolaryngol 2006;31:360–7.

59. Goodman MJ, Jhaveri M, Saverno K, et al. Cost-effectiveness of second-generation antihistamines and montelukast in relieving allergic rhinitis nasal symptoms. Am Health Drug Benefits 2008;1:26–34.

60. Badorrek P, Dick M, Schauerte A, et al. A combination of cetirizine and pseudoephedrine has therapeutic benefits when compared to single drug treatment in allergic rhinitis. Int J Clin Pharmacol Ther 2009;47:71–7.

61. Zieglmayer UP, Horak F, Toth J, et al. Efficacy and safety of an oral formulation of cetirizine and prolonged-release pseudoephedrine versus budesonide nasal spray in the management of nasal congestion in allergic rhinitis. Treat Respir Med 2005;4:283–7.

62. Meltzer EO, LaForce C, Ratner P, et al. MP29-02 (a novel intranasal formulation of azelastine hydrochloride and fluticasone propionate) in the treatment of seasonal allergic rhinitis: a randomized, double-blind, placebo-controlled trial of efficacy and safety. Allergy Asthma Proc 2012;33:324–32.

# Techniques in Septoplasty
## Traditional Versus Endoscopic Approaches

Janki Shah, MD, Christopher R. Roxbury, MD, Raj Sindwani, MD*

## KEYWORDS

- Septoplasty • Septal deviation • Endoscopic septoplasty • Open septoplasty
- Nasal obstruction

## KEY POINTS

- Surgical correction of a deviated septum can be addressed using the traditional open endonasal approach, the endoscopic approach, or the open septorhinoplasty approach.
- Thorough knowledge of the anatomy and physiology of the nose and sound operative technique are necessary to perform a successful septoplasty using either approach.
- Compared with the traditional open technique, the endoscopic septoplasty provides enhanced visualization of nasal anatomy and is particularly advantageous in addressing issues of the posterior septum.
- Caudal deformities are most readily addressed using open techniques.
- The location and severity of the septal deformity, along with surgeon experience and preference, play an important role in the selection of the septoplasty technique.

## INTRODUCTION

The nasal septum is an integral support structure of the nose. Deviation or deformity of the septum can cause nasal obstruction, the most common complaint in the average rhinologic practice.[1] If conservative medical management is unsuccessful in relieving symptoms of obstruction, surgical intervention to correct the septal deformity is indicated. Septoplasty is one of the most well-established and commonly performed procedures in otolaryngology. Although most often performed to fix structural deformities resulting in nasal obstruction, surgical correction of a deviated nasal septum may also be indicated in cases of recurrent epistaxis, sinusitis, obstructive sleep apnea, and facial pain/headaches secondary to septal spurs contacting the lateral nasal wall (Sluder syndrome). Additionally, septoplasty may be necessary for improved access during endoscopic sinus surgery (ESS), endoscopic orbital procedures (eg,

Disclosure Statement: The authors have no personal or financial conflicts of interest or disclosures regarding any of the material discussed within this article.
Head and Neck Institute, Cleveland Clinic, 9500 Euclid Avenue A71, Cleveland, OH 44195, USA
* Corresponding author.
E-mail address: sindwar@ccf.org

Otolaryngol Clin N Am 51 (2018) 909–917
https://doi.org/10.1016/j.otc.2018.05.007
0030-6665/18/

dacryocystorhinostomy, orbital decompression), and endoscopic endonasal skull base procedures.[2,3]

The 3 main approaches used to perform septoplasty include the traditional open endonasal approach, the recently popularized endoscopic approach, and the external open or open septorhinoplasty approach. First described by Freer[4] and Killian[5] in the early twentieth century, the traditional approach to address a deviated nasal septum involves direct visualization using headlight illumination and a nasal speculum. Alternatively, endoscopic septoplasty, which was initially described by Lanza and colleagues[6] and Stammberger[7] in 1991, involves the use of rigid endoscopes for visualization and targeted correction of any deformities. Both techniques can be used to address nasal septal deviations and have been shown to have similar functional outcomes.[8–11] The external open approach, which is often used to address markedly caudally deviated septa with accompanying external nasal deformities, is not discussed in this article.

## RELEVANT ANATOMY OF THE NASAL SEPTUM

A thorough understanding of the anatomy of the nasal septum is necessary when performing a septoplasty. The nasal septum has both functional and cosmetic significance and serves many purposes, including separating the nasal airway into 2 distinct cavities, providing dorsal support, maintaining the shape of the columella and nasal tip, and regulating airflow through the nose. Composed of membranous, cartilaginous, and osseous components, the nasal septum is the main support structure of the nose. The membranous septum, composed of fibrofatty tissue, is located anteriorly between the columellar lower lateral cartilages, whereas the cartilaginous septum, formed by the quadrangular cartilage, is just posterior to the membranous portion of the septum. The quadrangular cartilage has attachments to the upper and lower lateral cartilages anteriorly, the maxillary crest inferiorly, and the bony septum posteriorly. The osseous components of the septum include the vomer posteriorly, the perpendicular plate of the ethmoid postero-superiorly, and the nasal crest of the maxillary and palatine bones inferiorly. The perpendicular plate of the ethmoid bone is continuous with the cribriform plate superiorly and the sphenoid rostrum postero-superiorly, whereas the vomer fuses with the maxillary crest inferiorly (Fig. 1). Of note, the nasal septum forms the medial aspect of the internal nasal valve, the narrowest point of the nasal airway, where minute deviations in the septal structure can significantly affect airflow resistance and result in symptoms of nasal obstruction. The nasal septal swell body (or septal turbinate) is a normal, highly conserved component of the anterior nasal septum that should not be confused with a septal deviation. This mucosal-lined, fusiform swelling located anterior to the middle turbinate head and superior to the level of the inferior turbinate is readily identified on examination and imaging studies. Although little is known regarding its function, its anatomic location near the internal nasal valve and its histologic composition of both glandular and vasoerectile tissues suggest it may play a role in regulating nasal airflow.[12]

The nasal septum is lined with pseudostratified ciliated columnar respiratory epithelium along the inferior two-thirds and often contains olfactory epithelium along the superior one-third. The lateral surfaces of the septal cartilage and bones are covered with the mucoperichondrium and mucoperiosteum, respectively, which contain the blood supply and innervation of the septum. The nasal septum has a rich vascular supply originating from both the internal and external carotid arteries. The internal carotid artery supplies the septum via the anterior and posterior ethmoidal divisions of ophthalmic artery, which both course medially to traverse the roof of the nasal cavity

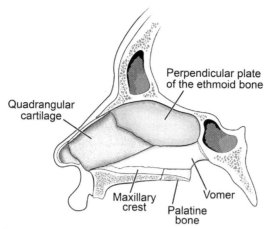

**Fig. 1.** Anatomy of nasal septum. (*Courtesy of* David Schumick, BS, CMI; with the permission of the Cleveland Clinic Center for Medical Art & Photography © 2018. All Rights Reserved.)

and supply the superior part of the nasal septum. The external carotid artery provides most of the blood supply to the nasal mucosa via terminal branches of the facial and internal maxillary arteries. The facial artery supplies the anterior septum via the septal branch of the superior labial artery, whereas the internal maxillary artery gives rise to the greater palatine artery, which supplies the inferior septum, and the sphenopalatine artery, which supplies most of the lateral nasal wall and posterior septum. Anastomoses of these arterial branches gives rise to the Kiesselbach plexus along the anterior septum bilaterally, a common site of epistaxis (**Fig. 2**). The trigeminal nerve (cranial nerve [CN] V) provides innervation to the nasal mucosa. The nasopalatine nerve, a branch of the maxillary nerve (CN V2), innervates the posteroinferior aspect of the nasal mucosa, whereas the anterior ethmoidal nerves, branches of the nasociliary

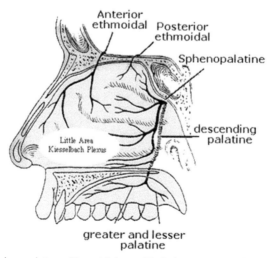

**Fig. 2.** Nasal septal vasculature. (*From* Viehweg TL, Roberson JB, Hudson JW. Epistaxis: diagnosis and treatment. J Oral Maxillofac Surg 2006;64(3):512; with permission.)

nerve from the ophthalmic nerve (CN VI), innervate the supero-anterior portion of the nasal mucosa. Superiorly, the olfactory nerve (CN I) provides innervation to the mucosa via small nerve endings that transverse the cribriform plate.[13]

## HISTORY OF SEPTOPLASTY

Surgery for correction of a deviated nasal septum has evolved over the course of many years. The first known accounts describing correction of nasal septal deformities can be found in ancient Egyptian medical literature dating as far back as 3500 BC. In the late nineteenth century, the Bosworth operation, which involved removing the deviation along with the overlying mucosa, was the most common procedure to correct nasal obstruction secondary to septal deviation.[14] Other early techniques discussed fracturing and splinting of the septum.[15]

In the early twentieth century, Killian[5] and Freer[4] described the submucous resection (SMR) operation, which has formed the foundation of modern septoplasty techniques. This technique involves raising the mucoperichondral flaps and resecting the cartilaginous and bony septum while leaving the overlying mucosa intact and leaving a 1-cm dorsal and 1-cm caudal segment, termed the L-strut, to maintain support (**Fig. 3**). The mucosal sparing technique, however, was less effective in correcting deviation of the caudal septum.[4,5] To address this, Metzenbaum[16] recommended the use of the swinging door technique in 1929, whereas Peer[17] advocated removing the caudal septum, straightening it, and then replacing it in the midline position in 1937. In 1948, Cottle and Loring[18] introduced the practice of conservative septal cartilage resections and replacement of bone and cartilage in the intramucosal space in an effort to avoid complications, including large septal perforations, saddle nose deformity, and columellar retraction, seen in patients who had undergone the SMR procedure and significant cartilage resection. More recently, Lanza and colleagues[6] and Stammberger[7] described endoscopic septoplasty, which has allowed septal pathologies to be addressed in a more directed fashion.

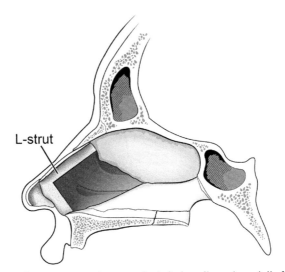

L-strut

**Fig. 3.** L-shaped cartilaginous strut that must be left dorsally and caudally for nasal support. (*Courtesy of* David Schumick, BS, CMI; with the permission of the Cleveland Clinic Center for Medical Art & Photography © 2018. All Rights Reserved.)

## TECHNIQUES IN SEPTOPLASTY

A cornerstone of the otolaryngologist's practice, septoplasty ranks as the third most common head and neck operation, with approximately 260,000 cases performed each year in the ambulatory setting.[19] The modern septoplasty has evolved into a more conservative procedure than the initially described SMR technique and involves resection of the targeted area of the deviated septum and may include modification and/or replacement of a cartilage graft. Despite its variations, each septoplasty technique is based on the fundamental principles of intact flap elevation, mucosal preservation, careful reapproximation, and preservation of dorsal and caudal supporting struts.

## TRADITIONAL SEPTOPLASTY

The traditional septoplasty is typically performed under general anesthesia using nasal speculums and headlight illumination for visualization. The nasal mucosa is decongested using topical epinephrine, oxymetazoline, or 4% cocaine. One percent lidocaine with 1:100,000 epinephrine is then injected along the septum bilaterally in a subperichondral plane in an anterior to posterior fashion until the mucosa is well blanched. The injection assists not only with local anesthesia and hemostasis but also with hydro-dissection. After allowing adequate time for vasoconstriction, either a Killian or hemi-transfixion incision is made using a 15 blade extending through the mucosa and perichondrium but sparing the cartilage itself. The side of the incision depends on surgeon preference. The Killian incision is placed approximately 1 to 2 cm posterior to the caudal septal margin and is useful when the septal deviation involves only the middle to posterior aspect of the septum. It does not provide adequate access to the anterior septum and is, thus, not used for caudal septal deviations. Alternatively, the hemi-transfixion incision, which is made at the caudal border of the septum, allows adequate exposure and is used when the caudal portion of the septum is involved. A curved elevator, such as the Cottle or Freer elevator, is then carefully used to dissect within a subperichondral plane and elevate the perichondrium and mucosa from the cartilage in an intact fashion. The dissection is continued broadly over and beyond the septal deformity, with care taken during flap elevation along the septal deviation or spur to avoid tearing the mucosa at these sites. Longer nasal speculums are used as needed throughout the procedure to ensure adequate visualization.

After the ipsilateral flap is elevated, the Cottle elevator or a 15 blade is used to gently incise the cartilage anterior to the site of the deviation and the contralateral flap is elevated. Care is taken to avoid tearing through the contralateral mucosa at the time of the cartilage incision and contralateral flap elevation to prevent septal perforation. Of note, an adequate L-strut is preserved to prevent loss of external nasal support and subsequent external deformity. Once both mucoperichondral flaps are elevated, the Cottle elevator, scissors, True-cut forceps, or Jansen Middleton forceps can be used to incise the cartilage superiorly and inferiorly to isolate the segment of deviated septum. The remaining deformity is then grasped using forceps, separated from its posterior attachment using a rotational movement in an anterior-posterior axis, and subsequently removed. It is important to ensure that the mucosa is not accidentally damaged when grasping the deviated segment. In addition, one must be careful to avoid a pulling or twisting motion outside of the anterior-posterior axis when maneuvering the deviated segment, as this could fracture the cribriform plate and result in a cerebrospinal fluid leak. Any remaining posterior bony deviation can be subsequently resected using True-cut or Jansen Middleton forceps. Of note, if the deviated segment of the septum is large, modifications of cartilage with cartilaginous scoring or weakening incisions can be used to minimize the extent of resected septal cartilage; alternatively, the removed cartilage can be morselized and replaced.

Once the septal deformity is resected, the mucoperichondral flaps are reapproximated and the initial mucosal incision is closed using an absorbable suture. A quilting stitch, nonabsorbable packing, or secured nasal splints are sometimes placed bilaterally to compress the flaps together. Patients are started on appropriate antibiotics with *Staphylococcus aureus* coverage as prophylaxis for toxic shock syndrome secondary to nasal packing. When used, the nasal packing or splints are removed in the clinic 3 to 5 days postoperatively.

## ENDOSCOPIC SEPTOPLASTY

Endoscopic septoplasty is very similar to the traditional approach. However, instead of a nasal speculum and headlight, rigid nasal endoscopes are used for illumination and visualization throughout the procedure. Often performed in conjunction with ESS, endoscopic septoplasty requires similar instrumentation and set up as these procedures. Under visualization using a $0°$ endoscope, the nasal mucosa is decongested and anesthetized as described with the traditional technique, and the location and severity of the septal deformity is examined. If the procedure is being performed for improved access and visualization before ESS, the position of the septum in relation to the middle turbinate is noted. A more posteriorly positioned modified Killian incision is made for complex or broad-based deviations, whereas a mucosal incision immediately anterior to or over the deformity is made for focal deviations or isolated septal spurs. Using a Cottle elevator, flaps are then elevated in a subperichondral or subperiosteal plane as previously described over the deviated cartilage or bone, with care taken to avoid mucosal tears in the area of thinned mucosa at the site of the deformity. The septal cartilage is then sharply incised, ensuring at least 1 cm of caudal and dorsal strut for nasal support. As described by Seth and colleagues,[20] the inferior turbinate concha and middle turbinate axilla are reliable landmarks; placing the mucosal incision at or posterior to the conchal line and at or inferior to the axillary line as defined in the study will result in adequate L-strut preservation. The mucoperichondral flap is then raised on the contralateral side, and the cartilaginous and/or osseous deformity is resected in a similar manner to that used in the traditional approach using a combination of True-cut, Jansen-Middleton, and Takahashi forceps. Some investigators have also described using the powered microdebrider to remove the deviated septum.[9,21,22] As with the nasal speculum in the traditional approach, the endoscope is used throughout the procedure in endoscopic septoplasty and can be placed between mucosal flaps and within the nasal cavity to ensure adequate resection of the septal deviation. Once this is completed, the mucosal flaps are repositioned and the mucosal incision and dead space created are closed with an absorbable suture. A quilting suture, nasal splints, or packing can be used as previously described to further reapproximate the flaps. It is worth mentioning that with the endoscopic approach, all steps of the operation described, from injection through incision and cartilage resection to suture placement, can be performed using the endoscope. A nasal speculum is not required.

## TRADITIONAL VERSUS ENDOSCOPIC APPROACH

Although studies[8–11] comparing endoscopic septoplasty with the traditional technique have shown similar patient outcomes, surgical results, and comparable operative times, the endoscopic technique offers several advantages over the open approach and may be indicated in certain clinical situations. By providing superior visualization of tissue planes with optimal illumination and magnification, the endoscopic approach allows the surgeon to more accurately evaluate the nasal anatomy and precisely and selectively remove the segments of the deviated septum. This ability is particularly useful in cases of isolated septal pathologies, such as distinct deviations or spurs that can be directly addressed. The endoscopic approach may also be helpful for submucoperichondral flap elevation during revision cases in which tissue planes are less obvious. In addition, the use of the endoscope may enhance the experience of residents and fellows and enables better teaching, as it projects the procedure onto a monitor. Limitations with the endoscopic technique have to do with the challenges of controlling the endoscope when operating very anteriorly in the nose where the nostril is not adequately available to support the endoscope (so-called free handing). For this reason, most surgeons consider caudal deflections a relative contraindication to the endoscopic technique and would favor open approaches in this clinical setting. Indications for the endoscopic approach, thus, include more posterior deviations of the septum without involvement of the caudal septum. In addition, as it is performed using similar instrumentation to ESS, endoscopic septoplasty can be performed in conjunction with ESS if necessary for improved access to the sinuses. Endoscopic septoplasty is contraindicated in cases of significant caudal deviations or a crooked nose, and the traditional open technique is preferred in cases of caudal septal deviations or severe septal deviations. Ultimately, the location and severity of the septal deformity along with surgeon experience and preference will play an important role in the selection of the septoplasty technique. Surgeons may opt to use a combined approach to take advantage of the unique benefits offered by each approach.

## COMPLICATIONS

Complications that can occur after septoplasty are nearly identical for both the traditional and endoscopic approaches. Persistent nasal obstruction is the most common complication, followed by septal perforation and external nasal deformity. Continuing sensation of nasal obstruction after surgery can be associated with incomplete repair of severe deviations, which require a more aggressive approach for correction. Septal perforations may result from unrepaired opposing mucoperichondral tears or can also occur as a result of vascular compromise of mucosa after postoperative hematoma or abscess. Overall, septal perforations are less likely to occur if mucosal flaps are kept intact during elevation. Risk of nasal deformities, such as tip ptosis or saddle nose deformity, which usually result from over-resection of the caudal septum or loss of dorsal nasal support, can be minimized by maintaining an adequate L-strut during septoplasty.[1–3,9,23]

Other complications can include epistaxis, septal hematoma, septal abscess, synechiae formation, and injury to the nasopalatine nerve with subsequent dental pain and hypesthesia. Although mild postoperative bleeding can occur, severe epistaxis after septoplasty is uncommon. Patients should be instructed to avoid the use of medications that can increase the risk of bleeding and to avoid strenuous activity and heavy lifting in the immediate postoperative period. Nasal packing, stents, and quilting sutures are thought to decrease the risk of postoperative bleeding and hematoma formation. Dental pain and hypesthesia can occur after septoplasty, but this is usually temporary and resolves within several weeks. Major complications, such as cerebrospinal fluid leak, unilateral blindness, and death, are extremely rare. In general, although some studies have reported reduced rates of certain complications, such as postoperative hemorrhage, mucosal adhesions, persistent deviation, and septal tears, with the endoscopic technique compared with the traditional approach, overall complication rates reported with endoscopic septoplasty are similar to those reported in the literature for traditional septoplasty.[9,23]

## SUMMARY

Surgical correction of a deviated septum can be performed using either the traditional open or endoscopic septoplasty techniques. Although both approaches have comparable outcomes and overall complication rates, the endoscopic approach offers certain advantages compared with traditional open septoplasty in appropriately selected patients. By providing enhanced visualization, the endoscopic technique allows the surgeon to more accurately examine nasal anatomy and directly address isolated septal pathologies with limited dissection. This visualization is also valuable for the education of residents and fellows. The endoscopic technique is also advantageous during ESS and during revision or complicated endoscopic cases, including pituitary and skull base procedures. Thorough knowledge of the anatomy and physiology of the nose and sound operative technique are necessary to perform a successful septoplasty using either approach. The location and severity of the septal deformity along with surgeon experience and preference play an important role in the selection of the septoplasty technique.

## REFERENCES

1. Konstantinidis I, Triaridis S, Triaridis A, et al. Long term results following nasal septal surgery, focus on patient satisfaction. Auris Nasus Larynx 2005;32:369–74.
2. Fettman N, Sanford T, Sindwani R. Surgical management of the deviated septum: techniques in septoplasty. Otolaryngol Clin North Am 2009;42(2):241–52, viii.
3. Sautter NB, Smith TL. Endoscopic septoplasty. Otolaryngol Clin North Am 2009; 42(2):253–60, viii.
4. Freer OT. The correction of deflections of the nasal septum with minimal traumatism. JAMA 1902;38:636–42.
5. Killian G. The submucous window resection of the nasal septum. Ann Otol Rhinol Laryngol 1905;14:363–93.
6. Lanza DC, Kennedy DW, Zinreich SJ. Nasal endoscopy and its surgical applications. In: Lee KJ, editor. Essential otolaryngology: head and neck surgery. 5th edition. New York: Medical Examination; 1991. p. 373–87.
7. Stammberger H. Special problems. In: Hawke M, editor. Functional endoscopic sinus surgery: the Messerklinger technique. Philadelphia: BC Decker; 1991. p. 432–3.
8. Chung BJ, Batra PS, Citardi MJ, et al. Endoscopic septoplasty: revisitation of the technique, indications, and outcomes. Am J Rhinol 2007;21:307–11.
9. Getz AE, Hwang PH. Endoscopic septoplasty. Curr Opin Otolaryngol Head Neck Surg 2008;16:26–31.
10. Hwang PH, McLaughlin RB, Lanza DC, et al. Endoscopic septoplasty: indications, technique, and results. Otolaryngol Head Neck Surg 1999;120:678–82.
11. Stewart M, Smith T, Weaver E, et al. Outcomes after nasal septoplasty: results from the nasal septoplasty effectiveness (NOSE) study. Otolaryngol Head Neck Surg 2004;130:283–90.
12. Costa D, Sanford T, Janney C, et al. Characterization of the nasal septal swell body. Arch Otolaryngol Head Neck Surg 2010;136(11):1107–10.

13. Kridel R, Sturm-O'Brien A. Nasal septum. In: Flint P, editor. Cummings otolaryngology–head & neck surgery. 6th edition. Philadelphia: Elsevier Saunders; 2015. p. 474–92.
14. Bailey B. Nasal septal surgery 1896–1899: transition and controversy. Laryngoscope 1997;107(1):10–6.
15. Adams W. The treatment of the broken nose by forcible straightening and mechanical apparatus. BMJ 1875;2:421–2.
16. Metzenbaum M. Replacement of the lower end of the dislocated septal cartilage versus submucous resection of the dislocated end of the septal cartilage. Arch Otolaryngol 1929;9:282–92.
17. Peer LA. An operation to repair lateral displacement of the lower border of the septal cartilage. Arch Otolaryngol 1937;25(4):475–7.
18. Cottle MH, Loring RM. Newer concepts of septum surgery: present status. Eye Ear Nose Throat Mon 1948;27:403–29.
19. Bhattacharyya N. Ambulatory sinus and nasal surgery in the United States: demographics and perioperative outcomes. Laryngoscope 2010;120(3):635–8.
20. Seth R, Haffey T, McBride JM, et al. Intranasal landmarks for adequate L-strut preservation during endoscopic septoplasty. Am J Rhinol Allergy 2014;28:265–8.
21. De Sousa A, Inciartef L, Levine H. Powered endoscopic nasal septal surgery. Acta Med Port 2005;18:249–56.
22. Raynor E. Powered endoscopic septoplasty for septal deviation and isolated spurs. Arch Facial Plast Surg 2005;7:410–2.
23. Hong CJ, Monteiro E, Badhiwala J, et al. Open versus endoscopic septoplasty techniques: a systematic review and meta-analysis. Am J Rhinol Allergy 2016; 30:436–42.

# Surgical Management of Turbinate Hypertrophy

Regan W. Bergmark, MD, Stacey T. Gray, MD*

## KEYWORDS

- Turbinate hypertrophy • Turbinates • Nasal obstruction • Turbinate reduction

## KEY POINTS

- Inferior turbinate reduction can be accomplished through a variety of techniques, such as submucosal resection, radiofrequency ablation, laser reduction surgery, and partial or complete turbinectomy approaches.
- Inferior turbinate reduction shows positive results in improving nasal obstruction symptoms postoperatively, but efficacy may decrease over time.
- Bleeding and crusting are the most common complications of turbinate surgery.
- Empty nose syndrome is a rare but morbid complication that is generally associated with significant removal of the inferior turbinate.
- High-quality clinical trials comparing techniques and assessing long-term outcomes are largely lacking; more research is needed.

## OVERVIEW AND HISTORICAL PERSPECTIVE

Turbinate surgery for nasal obstruction generally involves reducing the size of the inferior turbinate. Turbinate surgery has been a common otolaryngologic procedure since the late 1800s.[1] Initially, total inferior turbinectomy was advocated. This typically involved medializing the inferior turbinate and using a scissors or blade to fully resect the turbinate. Due to complications, such as bleeding, significant crusting, and atrophic rhinitis, and concerns about nonphysiologic air turbulence, total turbinectomy was largely abandoned. More recently, turbinate reduction procedures have been advocated and a variety of surgical options have been developed.[1]

---

Disclosure Statement: The authors did not receive financial support specifically for this project, but all authors have academic research grant funding for their other work. Dr R.W. Bergmark has research grant funding from the American Board of Medical Specialties Visiting Scholars Program and the Gliklich Healthcare Innovation Scholars Program. Dr S.T. Gray has no disclosures.
Department of Otolaryngology–Head and Neck Surgery, Massachusetts Eye and Ear, 243 Charles Street, Boston, MA 02114, USA
* Corresponding author.
*E-mail address:* Stacey_Gray@MEEI.Harvard.edu

Otolaryngol Clin N Am 51 (2018) 919–928
https://doi.org/10.1016/j.otc.2018.05.008
0030-6665/18/© 2018 Elsevier Inc. All rights reserved.

oto.theclinics.com

The inferior turbinate is composed of the bony turbinate, the submucosal tissue and the overlying mucosa. Surgical procedures involve resecting, ablating or crushing part, or all, of the turbinate to increase the size of the nasal airway. The appropriate choice of procedure may depend on a patient's anatomy and other concurrent procedures performed (such as septoplasty or septorhinoplasty) as well as the presence or absence of other comorbidities such as allergic rhinitis. A clinical consensus statement from the American Academy of Otolaryngology–Head and Neck Surgery on septoplasty with or without inferior turbinate reduction states that (1) "inferior turbinate hypertrophy can be an independent cause of nasal obstruction in the septoplasty patient" and (2) "inferior turbinoplasty is an effective adjunctive procedure to septoplasty for patients with inferior turbinate hypertrophy."[2] In regard to patients with inferior turbinate hypertrophy and allergic rhinitis, the American Academy of Otolaryngology Head and Neck Surgery clinical practice guidelines on allergic rhinitis state that "clinicians may offer inferior turbinate reduction in patients with [allergic rhinitis] with nasal airway obstruction and enlarged inferior turbinates who have failed medical management."[3]

## EFFICACY AND OUTCOMES MEASUREMENT OF INFERIOR TURBINATE REDUCTION SURGERY

Efficacy is best evaluated through patient reported outcomes measures. The Nasal Obstruction Symptom Evaluation instrument and visual analog scales are frequently used. Quantitative measures of nasal airflow, resistance, or volume do not necessarily correlate well with patient perception of effectiveness. Importantly, long-term follow-up after turbinate surgery is needed to further quantify surgical effectiveness; unfortunately, long-term outcomes are frequently lacking in the published literature (see Emily Spataro and Sam P. Most's article, "Measuring Nasal Obstruction Outcomes," in this issue, for more information on measurement of outcomes of turbinate surgery and other nasal obstruction treatment).

## COMPLICATIONS OF TURBINATE REDUCTION SURGERY

Major complications of inferior turbinate surgery are rare. Failure of the procedure to resolve nasal obstruction, either in the near term or long term, is the most common issue. Bleeding and crusting are the most frequently described complications. These complications have been reported more frequently with more aggressive techniques that include greater resection of the turbinate or surgery in the more posterior aspect of the turbinate, given the origin of the blood supply posteriorly. Bone necrosis, synechiae, anosmia, and atrophic rhinitis have been described but are rare and generally associated with more aggressive procedures.[1] Empty nose syndrome is a rare complication associated with turbinate surgery and is discussed more thoroughly later.

## LIMITED RANDOMIZED CONTROLLED TRIALS COMPARING TECHNIQUES

Randomized clinical trials with robust study design are largely lacking for inferior turbinate surgery despite the use of this technique for more than 120 years. Therefore, the authors are largely unable to draw comparative conclusions about the benefits and drawbacks of specific techniques and thus offer an overview of the different procedures available with some common advantages and drawbacks for each technique. A Cochrane review in 2010 did not find any studies that met inclusion criteria of randomized controlled trials comparing inferior turbinate surgical techniques or comparing inferior turbinate surgery to medical management of turbinate hypertrophy.[4] The main problems with existing studies that did not meet Cochrane inclusion criteria included lack of randomization, lack of long-term follow-up, lack of disease specificity (ie, combining allergic and nonallergic rhinitis patients), combining adult and pediatric patients, and small sample size.

From a value standpoint, there are insufficient published data on cost differences between techniques to make a recommendation on the most financially responsible approach. The equipment costs are different (ie, laser, microdébrider, simple blade, and radiofrequency ablation device) and may depend on the use of those tools by the surgeon and facility or hospital for other cases or within the same case for other portions of the procedure. Laser inferior turbinate surgery, for example, was written about extensively in the 1990s, with the purported benefits that it could be performed in the office without general anesthesia. Costly laser equipment, however, was needed.[5] For inferior turbinate reduction with septoplasty, there is significant cost variability based on surgeon, facility, operative time, equipment needs, and associated complications.[6] Future studies examining the costs of inferior turbinate reduction in isolation, and when bundled with other procedures, would help determine value for this specific component of the procedure.[6]

## TURBINOPLASTY AND PARTIAL TURBINECTOMY

Partial turbinectomy has been described with multiple different techniques, such as cold resection of part of the turbinate. Many techniques leave a portion of the anterior head for nasal humidification and the posterior aspect to decrease the risk of bleeding. Medial flap turbinoplasty has been described as a way to reduce the turbinate size with preservation of mucosa. The medial mucosal flap is elevated and left intact and the turbinate bone and lateral mucosa are resected. The branches of the inferior turbinate artery must be cauterized during this procedure. Good long-term results have been described with this technique although more studies are needed.[7]

## SUBMUCOSAL INFERIOR TURBINATE REDUCTION
### Technique

Submucosal resection involves preservation of the mucosa and bone with reduction of the submucosal tissue. Multiple techniques exist; a common technique involves using a number 15 blade to make an incision in the anterior head of the inferior turbinate and then a powered instrument, such as a small microdébrider can be introduced to resect the submucosa. The theory behind submucosal resection is that it preserves ciliary function and mucociliary clearance by protecting the mucosa but removes the tissue that is hypertrophied and leads to nasal obstruction.

### Evidence Base

Submucosal resection with powered instrumentation rarely has been studied in the absence of concurrent procedures. Good long-term results have been demonstrated in small studies,[8] and other studies have shown good results when combined with turbinate lateralization,[9] but more research is needed.

## LASER INFERIOR TURBINATE REDUCTION
### Technique

Various lasers have been used for turbinate reduction. $CO_2$, diode, Ho:YAG, Nd:YAG, argon-ion, and potassium titanyl phosphate (KTP) laser systems have been described in the literature. Laser turbinate reduction has been described with many different techniques, such as contact, noncontact, or interstitial. Lasers have been described in the operating room and in the outpatient clinic setting with topical anesthesia.

### Evidence Base

Laser turbinate reduction was popularized in the 1990s, with a proliferation of research during that time, and less so in the past 10 years. One review stated that laser turbinate reduction could be done in the outpatient setting under local anesthesia but was generally less effective long term compared with submucosal resection, turbinoplasty (partial reduction), or turbinectomy.[10] Some investigators have described good long-term results with relief of nasal obstruction in a majority of patients at 2 years to 5 years postoperatively.[11,12] Other investigators have likewise endorsed good effectiveness of laser inferior turbinate reduction as long as the nasal obstruction is due to swollen soft tissue of the interior turbinate.[13] No high-quality studies demonstrate significant differences in techniques that would lead to a strong recommendation for a specific laser type. In 1 comparison between laser types, there were no statistically significant differences in outcomes, with approximately half of patients reporting subjective improvement at 1 year.[14] The varying lasers do have different tissue penetration and field effects. For example, $CO_2$ laser has a more narrow field effect with more targeted effects but also a higher potential risk for bleeding complications than other lasers discussed in this article.[15] One study showed that 84% of patients who underwent diode laser inferior turbinate reduction surgery had improvement of symptoms at 1 year.[16]

## INFERIOR TURBINATE OUTFRACTURE
### Technique

Outfracture of the inferior turbinate is accomplished by compressing the inferior turbinate laterally or inferolaterally until the bony turbinate fractures. It is generally accomplished with a blunt instrument, such as a Boise elevator or Freer elevator. Some surgeons infracture the turbinate first (pull the inferior aspect of the turbinate medially) prior to outfracture of the turbinate.

### Evidence Base

Inferior turbinate outfracture is commonly used during nasal surgeries with minimal side effects but generally has not shown lasting duration of symptomatic improvement. In many studies, it appears the turbinate either remedializes or continues to hypertrophy such that benefit is lost. Therefore, turbinate outfracture is generally used in combination with an additional technique to improve nasal airflow, such as turbinate reduction or septoplasty.[17]

A recent study showed that after outfracture, the bony turbinate remains lateralized at 6 months postoperatively, but that the overlying soft tissue hypertrophies in a compensatory fashion.[18] CT scans were performed preoperatively and 6 months postoperatively on patients. The distance to the inferior turbinate bone from the median line increased, showing that the turbinate bone remained lateralized; the width of the bone was also smaller.[18] The soft tissue of the inferior turbinate increased, however, between preoperative and postoperative CT scans, demonstrating compensatory hypertrophy.[18] The investigators concluded that a volume reduction surgery should be performed in addition to outfracture.[18]

## RADIOFREQUENCY INFERIOR TURBINATE REDUCTION
### Technique

Radiofrequency volumetric tissue reduction (RFVTR) of the inferior turbinate is one of the most common methods of reducing the soft tissue component of the turbinate. Monopolar or bipolar radiofrequency can be used; newer radiofrequency techniques have also been tested. A long, sharp turbinate blade for the monopolar can be used, which is inserted into the inferior turbinate and turned on to reduce the inferior turbinate submucosal tissue while attempting to spare the majority of the mucosal surface. Other techniques include direct application of the monopolar or bipolar to the external turbinate rather than through a submucosal application.

### Evidence Base

Studies generally demonstrate short-term improvement, with more limited studies on long-term follow-up. A randomized clinical trial with 22 patients with a crossover design demonstrated short-term superiority of bipolar radiofrequency ablation compared with placebo 6 weeks to 8 weeks after intervention.[19] A study of 40 patients undergoing radiofrequency inferior turbinate reduction demonstrated improvement of symptoms as well as odor thresholds at 2 years postoperatively.[20] Improvement in patient-reported outcome measures and objective measures of nasal airflow has also been demonstrated 3 years from time of treatment.[21] At 3 years, a majority of patients undergoing RFVTR showed some sustained reduction in symptoms, although patients with allergic rhinitis had a greater likelihood of symptom relapse versus those without allergic rhinitis.[22] Ciliary function and mucociliary clearance are generally preserved long term with this technique. For example, in 1 study, ciliary function returned to normal by 3 months after radiofrequency ablation, and no changes were noted in mucociliary clearance in an even shorter time frame (1 month, 2 months, or 3 months).[23]

### Differences in Type of Radiofrequency

One randomized single-blind study between bipolar and monopolar radiofrequency ablation showed no difference at 6 months in level of improvement, although in the first week, the monopolar group had more symptomatic relief and less pain. Overall, the monopolar was used for greater treatment duration than the bipolar.[24] One randomized study on temperature-controlled radiofrequency versus bipolar radiofrequency found no difference in outcomes at 1 year, but the bipolar procedure was faster.[25] A new radiofrequency method, quantic molecular resonance, has also recently been described,[26] but needs to be compared with other turbinate reduction techniques. A randomized noncontrolled study comparing radiofrequency turbinate volume reduction versus radiofrequency assisted turbinate resection demonstrated improvements in symptoms at 6 months postoperatively that were similar between groups but more adverse events and slightly higher postoperative morbidity in the turbinate resection group.[27]

## INFERIOR TURBINATE REDUCTION: OTHER TECHNIQUES

Other techniques for inferior turbinate reduction or resection have been described. Coblation has been studied in short-term studies.[28] Cryotherapy and ultrasound-assisted reduction have also been described.[17,29]

## TECHNIQUE COMPARISON

A recent Cochrane review[4] found no randomized controlled trials up through mid-2010 meeting the criteria for inclusion. Subsequently, a brief literature review published in the *Laryngoscope* in 2013[28] examined 5 prospective randomized trials.[9,30–33] All 5 studies were completed and published prior to the Cochrane review, and none met the more stringent Cochrane study guidelines for inclusion. The *Laryngoscope* article concluded, "submucosal resection combined with lateral displacement is the most effective at decreasing nasal obstruction caused by inferior turbinate hypertrophy. In the turbinoplasty group, based on the current evidence, microdebrider-assisted and ultrasound turbinate reduction have been shown to be the most effective. A prospective randomized trial comparing the microdebrider assisted and ultrasound turbinate reduction has not yet been performed."[28] Overall, technique decisions are often made based on decision to perform the procedure in the office or in the operating room, concurrent with other procedures, cost, potential complications, surgeon familiarity, and comfort.[34] More studies are needed to determine if there are clinically significant differences in long-term outcomes or complications based on technique.[34]

### Microdébrider Versus Radiofrequency

A 2015 meta-analysis comparing radiofrequency ablation with microdébrider inferior turbinate reduction found that both techniques were effective in improving visual analog scale–rated nasal obstruction and acoustic rhinomanometry results, but median follow-up was only 6 months.[35] They demonstrated no significant differences in outcomes based on technique.[35] That study focused on the primary outcome measures of a visual analog scale for nasal obstruction and secondary outcomes measure of acoustic rhinomanometry results (study size range, N = 7–197). On their quality-assessment scale of 0 to 3 (3 is best quality), the mean study score was 1.35 (median 1.0).

### Medial Flap Turbinoplasty Versus Submucosal Electrocautery

Medial flap turbinoplasty is a method to reduce turbinate volume while protecting the turbinate mucosa.[7] A randomized controlled trial of patients undergoing submucosal powered tissue reduction with either submucosal electrocautery or medial flap turbinoplasty stated that the medial flap turbinoplasty produced the best long-term results at 60 months, whereas electrocautery produced the most postoperative crusting.[36]

### Laser Versus Radiofrequency

One study raised the concern that mucociliary clearance was significantly disturbed with $CO_2$ laser ablation compared with radiofrequency tissue ablation and partial turbinectomy at 12 weeks postoperatively, although the study was small.[37] A separate study of inferior turbinate reduction in a pig model showed that although Nd:YAG and KTP laser reduction as well as radiofrequency tissue reduction techniques all had functional cilia and volume reduction at 6 weeks after the procedure, there were more histopathologic healing complications associated with the 2 laser groups, such as dilated mucus glands.[38] Radiofrequency treatment and diode laser had similar efficacy at 3 months in another small, randomized trial.[39] Patients had more intraoperative discomfort with the radiofrequency treatment and yet more patients said they would choose that treatment in the future.[39]

### Coblation Versus Other Techniques

In 1 comparison, radiofrequency ablation and coblation were found equally effective in the short term, but their effectiveness diminished by 3 years.[40] Coblation and microdébrider inferior turbinate reduction were equivalent in short-term outcomes in another study, with significant inferior turbinate size reduction and reduction in nasal obstruction symptoms. The coblation group also had less postoperative pain.[41]

## INFERIOR TURBINATE REDUCTION WITH SEPTORHINOPLASTY

The benefit of inferior turbinate reduction concurrent with septorhinoplasty is unclear, and more rigorous and larger randomized controlled trials are needed. A recent randomized clinical trial of 50 patients comparing partial inferior turbinate resection (posterior one-third) versus no turbinate surgery during functional septorhinoplasty found no changes in general or disease-specific quality-of-life outcomes or complications between patients in the 2 groups. Operative times were significantly longer in the turbinate surgery group (212 minutes vs 159 minutes).[42] Another randomized clinical trial found no difference between septorhinoplasty alone and septorhinoplasty with inferior turbinate reduction in quality of life and acoustic rhinomanometry findings at 3 months, although fewer patients who had undergone turbinate reduction were on topical intranasal corticosteroids.[43] Nasal obstruction concerns during septorhinoplasty are discussed further in Douglas Sidle and Katherine Hicks's article, "Nasal Obstruction Considerations in Cosmetic Rhinoplasty," in this issue.

## INFERIOR TURBINATE SURGERY AND OTOLOGIC SYMPTOMS (EUSTACHIAN TUBE DYSFUNCTION)

The anterior head of the inferior turbinate, which is believed to contribute most substantially to nasal obstruction symptoms, does not seem to drive otologic symptoms. A recent randomized placebo (sham procedure)-controlled clinical trial of the effect of turbinate surgery on eustachian tube dysfunction problems found no significant differences between groups.[44] Patients undergoing turbinate surgery, as well as patients undergoing a sham procedure, had significant improvements in the Eustachian Tube Dysfunction Questionnaire scores. Patients in the intervention group underwent microdébrider surgery, diode laser, or radiofrequency ablation of the anterior half of the turbinate. Tympanometry was not different between groups at 3 months. Therefore, the study did "not support the use of reduction of the anterior half of the inferior turbinate as the sole procedure intended to treat ear symptoms."[44] More studies are needed, particularly with attention to techniques addressing the posterior half of the inferior turbinate.

## EMPTY NOSE SYNDROME

Empty nose syndrome is a rare condition in which patients have substantial subjective nasal obstruction despite significant space for airflow in the nasal cavity. Empty nose syndrome almost exclusively seen in patients who have had turbinate surgery and is classically described as a complication of complete resection of the inferior turbinates. It is associated with reduced inferior turbinate volume, when comparing patients with this condition to control patients (patients who had undergone pituitary adenoma resection and did not have empty nose syndrome).[45] It was the reason, however, why less aggressive approaches to inferior turbinate resection became more popular.

A recent study on 6 patients with empty nose syndrome found that nasal airflow was streamlined and jetlike in the middle meatus region, with limited airflow in the region of the inferior turbinates.[46] The authors also found evidence of potential sensory impairment, with reduced trigeminal nerve function as evidenced by impaired lateral detection tests of menthol.[46]

## SUMMARY

Although a large number of published articles exist on turbinate reduction or resection, high-quality randomized clinical trials are limited. Submucosal resection, radiofrequency ablation, laser reduction, and limited resection are the most commonly described techniques, without sufficient long-term data to make strong recommendations between them. Inferior turbinate outfracture alone seems ineffective. Total resection of the inferior turbinate should not be performed for nasal obstruction, based on a small but real risk of empty nose syndrome. More long-term studies are needed to determine long-term efficacy and to distinguish any clinically significant differences in outcomes between techniques.

## REFERENCES

1. Nurse LA, Duncavage JA. Surgery of the inferior and middle turbinates. Otolaryngol Clin North Am 2009;42(2):295–309, ix.
2. Han JK, Stringer SP, Rosenfeld RM, et al. Clinical consensus statement: septoplasty with or without inferior turbinate reduction. Otolaryngol Head Neck Surg 2015;153(5):708–20.
3. Seidman MD, Gurgel RK, Lin SY, et al. Clinical practice guideline: allergic rhinitis. Otolaryngol Head Neck Surg 2015;152(1 Suppl):S1–43.
4. Jose J, Coatesworth AP. Inferior turbinate surgery for nasal obstruction in allergic rhinitis after failed medical treatment. Cochrane Database Syst Rev 2010;(12):CD005235.
5. Englender M. Nasal laser mucotomy (L-mucotomy) of the interior turbinates. J Laryngol Otol 1995;109(4):296–9.
6. Thomas A, Alt J, Gale C, et al. Surgeon and hospital cost variability for septoplasty and inferior turbinate reduction. Int Forum Allergy Rhinol 2016;6(10):1069–74.
7. Barham HP, Knisely A, Harvey RJ, et al. How I do it: medial flap inferior turbinoplasty. Am J Rhinol Allergy 2015;29(4):314–5.
8. Yanez C, Mora N. Inferior turbinate debriding technique: ten-year results. Otolaryngol Head Neck Surg 2008;138(2):170–5.
9. Passali D, Passali FM, Damiani V, et al. Treatment of inferior turbinate hypertrophy: a randomized clinical trial. Ann Otol Rhinol Laryngol 2003;112(8):683–8.
10. Janda P, Sroka R, Baumgartner R, et al. Laser treatment of hyperplastic inferior nasal turbinates: a review. Lasers Surg Med 2001;28(5):404–13.
11. Katz S, Schmelzer B, Vidts G. Treatment of the obstructive nose by CO2-laser reduction of the inferior turbinates: technique and results. Am J Rhinol 2000; 14(1):51–5.
12. Lagerholm S, Harsten G, Emgard P, et al. Laser-turbinectomy: long-term results. J Laryngol Otol 1999;113(6):529–31.
13. Lippert BM, Werner JA. Long-term results after laser turbinectomy. Lasers Surg Med 1998;22(2):126–34.
14. DeRowe A, Landsberg R, Leonov Y, et al. Subjective comparison of Nd:YAG, diode, and CO2 lasers for endoscopically guided inferior turbinate reduction surgery. Am J Rhinol 1998;12(3):209–12.
15. Janda P, Sroka R, Betz CS, et al. Comparison of laser induced effects on hyperplastic inferior nasal turbinates by means of scanning electron microscopy. Lasers Surg Med 2002;30(1):31–9.
16. Cakli H, Cingi C, Guven E, et al. Diode laser treatment of hypertrophic inferior turbinates and evaluation of the results with acoustic rhinometry. Eur Arch Otorhinolaryngol 2012;269(12):2511–7.
17. Sinno S, Mehta K, Lee ZH, et al. Inferior turbinate hypertrophy in rhinoplasty: systematic review of surgical techniques. Plast Reconstr Surg 2016;138(3): 419e–29e.

18. Lee DC, Jin SG, Kim BY, et al. Does the effect of inferior turbinate outfracture persist? Plast Reconstr Surg 2017;139(2):386e–91e.

19. Bran GM, Hunnebeck S, Herr RM, et al. Bipolar radiofrequency volumetric tissue reduction of the inferior turbinates: evaluation of short-term efficacy in a prospective, randomized, single-blinded, placebo-controlled crossover trial. Eur Arch Otorhinolaryngol 2013;270(2):595–601.

20. Garzaro M, Pezzoli M, Landolfo V, et al. Radiofrequency inferior turbinate reduction: long-term olfactory and functional outcomes. Otolaryngol Head Neck Surg 2012;146(1):146–50.

21. Assanasen P, Banhiran W, Tantilipikorn P, et al. Combined radiofrequency volumetric tissue reduction and lateral outfracture of hypertrophic inferior turbinate in the treatment of chronic rhinitis: short-term and long-term outcome. Int Forum Allergy Rhinol 2014;4(4):339–44.

22. De Corso E, Bastanza G, Di Donfrancesco V, et al. Radiofrequency volumetric inferior turbinate reduction: long-term clinical results. Acta Otorhinolaryngol Ital 2016;36(3):199–205.

23. Rosato C, Pagliuca G, Martellucci S, et al. Effect of radiofrequency thermal ablation treatment on nasal ciliary motility: a study with phase-contrast microscopy. Otolaryngol Head Neck Surg 2016;154(4):754–8.

24. Kocak HE, Altas B, Aydin S, et al. Assessment of inferior turbinate radiofrequency treatment: Monopolar versus bipolar. Otolaryngol Pol 2016;70(4):22–8.

25. Banhiran W, Assanasen P, Tantilipikorn P, et al. A randomized study of temperature-controlled versus bipolar radiofrequency for inferior turbinate reduction. Eur Arch Otorhinolaryngol 2015;272(10):2877–84.

26. Di Rienzo Businco L, Di Rienzo Businco A, Ventura L, et al. Turbinoplasty with quantic molecular resonance in the treatment of persistent moderate-severe allergic rhinitis: Comparative analysis of efficacy. Am J Rhinol Allergy 2014; 28(2):164–8.

27. Kumar S, Anand TS, Pal I. Radiofrequency turbinate volume reduction vs. radiofrequency-assisted turbinectomy for nasal obstruction caused by inferior turbinate hypertrophy. Ear Nose Throat J 2017;96(2):e23–6.

28. Larrabee YC, Kacker A. Which inferior turbinate reduction technique best decreases nasal obstruction? Laryngoscope 2014;124(4):814–5.

29. Bhattacharyya N, Kepnes LJ. Clinical effectiveness of coblation inferior turbinate reduction. Otolaryngol Head Neck Surg 2003;129(4):365–71.

30. Nease CJ, Krempl GA. Radiofrequency treatment of turbinate hypertrophy: a randomized, blinded, placebo-controlled clinical trial. Otolaryngol Head Neck Surg 2004;130(3):291–9.

31. Gindros G, Kantas I, Balatsouras DG, et al. Comparison of ultrasound turbinate reduction, radiofrequency tissue ablation and submucosal cauterization in inferior turbinate hypertrophy. Eur Arch Otorhinolaryngol 2010;267(11): 1727–33.

32. Cingi C, Ure B, Cakli H, et al. Microdebrider-assisted versus radiofrequency-assisted inferior turbinoplasty: a prospective study with objective and subjective outcome measures. Acta Otorhinolaryngol Ital 2010;30(3):138–43.

33. Liu CM, Tan CD, Lee FP, et al. Microdebrider-assisted versus radiofrequency-assisted inferior turbinoplasty. Laryngoscope 2009;119(2):414–8.

34. Brunworth J, Holmes J, Sindwani R. Inferior turbinate hypertrophy: review and graduated approach to surgical management. Am J Rhinol Allergy 2013;27(5): 411–5.

35. Acevedo JL, Camacho M, Brietzke SE. Radiofrequency ablation turbinoplasty versus microdebrider-assisted turbinoplasty: a systematic review and meta-analysis. Otolaryngol Head Neck Surg 2015;153(6):951–6.

36. Barham HP, Thornton MA, Knisely A, et al. Long-term outcomes in medial flap inferior turbinoplasty are superior to submucosal electrocautery and submucosal powered turbinate reduction. Int Forum Allergy Rhinol 2016;6(2):143–7.

37. Sapci T, Sahin B, Karavus A, et al. Comparison of the effects of radiofrequency tissue ablation, CO2 laser ablation, and partial turbinectomy applications on nasal mucociliary functions. Laryngoscope 2003;113(3):514–9.

38. Somogyvari K, Moricz P, Gerlinger I, et al. Morphological and histological effects of radiofrequency and laser (KTP and Nd:YAG) treatment of the inferior turbinates in animals. Surg Innov 2017;24(1):5–14.

39. Kisser U, Stelter K, Gurkov R, et al. Diode laser versus radiofrequency treatment of the inferior turbinate - a randomized clinical trial. Rhinology 2014;52(4):424–30.

40. Passali D, Loglisci M, Politi L, et al. Managing turbinate hypertrophy: coblation vs. radiofrequency treatment. Eur Arch Otorhinolaryngol 2016;273(6):1449–53.

41. Hegazy HM, ElBadawey MR, Behery A. Inferior turbinate reduction; coblation versus microdebrider - a prospective, randomised study. Rhinology 2014;52(4):306–14.

42. de Moura BH, Migliavacca RO, Lima RK, et al. Partial inferior turbinectomy in rhinoseptoplasty has no effect in quality-of-life outcomes: a randomized clinical trial. Laryngoscope 2018;128(1):57–63.

43. Lavinsky-Wolff M, Camargo HL Jr, Barone CR, et al. Effect of turbinate surgery in rhinoseptoplasty on quality-of-life and acoustic rhinometry outcomes: a randomized clinical trial. Laryngoscope 2013;123(1):82–9.

44. Harju T, Kivekas I, Numminen J, et al. The effect of inferior turbinate surgery on ear symptoms. Laryngoscope 2018;128(3):568–72.

45. Hong HR, Jang YJ. Correlation between remnant inferior turbinate volume and symptom severity of empty nose syndrome. Laryngoscope 2016;126(6):1290–5.

46. Li C, Farag AA, Leach J, et al. Computational fluid dynamics and trigeminal sensory examinations of empty nose syndrome patients. Laryngoscope 2017;127(6):e176–84.

# Surgical Management of Nasal Valve Collapse

Sheena Samra, MD, Jeffrey T. Steitz, MD, Natalia Hajnas, BA,
Dean M. Toriumi, MD*

## KEYWORDS

- Internal and external nasal valve • Nasal valve collapse • Nasal obstruction
- Nasal valve repair

## KEY POINTS

- Nasal valve collapse is a common cause of nasal obstruction and is oftentimes iatrogenic due to previous reductive rhinoplasty.
- Nonsurgical methods of management exist, and newly designed implants can significantly improve lateral wall and nasal valve collapse.
- Surgical management of the nasal valve is focused primarily on widening the valve and providing support to the lateral wall with appropriate autologous grafting techniques.

## INTRODUCTION

Nasal valve collapse is a common cause of functional upper airway obstruction that leads to varying difficulty with nasal inspiration, diminished exercise tolerance, and significant decreases in quality of life. Nasal valve collapse can be innate to patient anatomy, iatrogenic, congenital, or traumatic, but regardless of cause, causes significant patient distress.

The nasal valve can be subdivided into internal and external components. The internal nasal valve refers to the area defined by the nasal septum medially, the upper lateral cartilages superolaterally, and the head of the inferior turbinate inferiorly. The cross-sectional area of the nasal ala, or opening of the nasal vestibule, defines the external nasal valve.[1] The muscles responsible for maintaining nasal valve patency during inspiration include the nasalis and dilator naris muscles. Both muscles prevent nasal valve collapse on deep inspiration by acting directly on the upper lateral cartilages and alar soft tissue.[2] Furthermore, the nasal valve provides the greatest resistance to airflow in the nose and, when compromised, can lead to nasal valve

Disclosure Statement: D.M. Toriumi - Spirox Latera implant – Consultant. The other authors have nothing to disclose.
Department of Otolaryngology, Head and Neck Surgery, University of Illinois at Chicago, 60 East, Delaware, Suite 1411, Chicago, IL 606114, USA
* Corresponding author.
E-mail address: dtoriumi@uic.edu

Otolaryngol Clin N Am 51 (2018) 929–944
https://doi.org/10.1016/j.otc.2018.05.009
0030-6665/18/Published by Elsevier Inc.

oto.theclinics.com

collapse with significant functional deficiencies with worsened quality of life. As the airflow increases through the nasal valves, negative pressure is produced, which leads to collapse of the nasal valve and lateral wall. Because of velocity of airflow inherently creating negative pressure within the nasal valve, iatrogenic narrowing or loss of lateral wall support reliably leads to significant supra-alar pinching and eventual obstruction.

Rhinoplasty is the most common cause of nasal valve dysfunction.[2] In a study series of 100 secondary rhinoplasty cases, Constantian[2] found that 50% of patients endorsed external nasal valve obstruction and 645 of patients complained of nasal obstruction at the internal valve.[1] Overresection of the upper lateral cartilages, excessive narrowing of the dorsum, and displacement of short nasal bones correlate with internal nasal valve obstruction. Aggressive narrowing of the nasal tip, overresection of lateral crura, and displacement of weak alar cartilages correlate with external nasal valve obstruction. Although patients may not experience severe obstruction in the immediate postoperative period, negative pressure through the nasal airway will lead to eventual displacement of the lateral wall medially leading to a worse cosmetic appearance and significant functional obstruction that may require revision surgery.

Nasal valve clinical assessment includes not only history taking for likely etiologic causes but also a thorough physical examination. Assessing patient nasal airflow at rest and on inspiration is paramount to determine the presence and severity of nasal valve collapse. The Cottle maneuver, which is a lateral distraction of the cheek away from the airway, is a rather nonspecific test and almost uniformly shows improvement in breathing without specificity for site of obstruction.[2] The authors prefer the use of a wire loop curette to stent the lateral crus, which is the most common location of lateral wall collapse (modified Cottle maneuver). In regards to external nasal valve compromise, there are several physical examination findings often noted: thin skin, deep supra-alar groove, parenthesis deformity of tip, narrow nostrils with overprojection of the tip, short medial crus with associated widened columella, and caudal septal deviation with contralateral external nasal valve collapse on deep inspiration.[3] With cephalically malpositioned lateral crura, there may be a bulbous tip and alar retraction, which also manifest as external nasal valve collapse. The cephalic positioning of the lateral crura leaves the lateral wall of the nose void of cartilage support, potentially resulting in collapse upon inspiration.

Defining the degree of nasal obstruction is an important outcome measure. The NOSE questionnaire, a validated quality-of-life assessment instrument, allows standardization of the symptoms of nasal obstruction in assessing functional improvements.[4] The questionnaire comprises 5 questions to better understand their nasal obstruction and is a powerful adjunct, but does not supplant a good history and physical examination.

Once a diagnosis of nasal valve collapse is made and the cause is determined, appropriate management can be discussed with the patient. There are several nonsurgical options as well as a wide array of surgical maneuvers to improve nasal valve collapse. Nonsurgical management focuses on stenting or providing external support to the nasal valve and lateral wall. Surgical maneuvers focus more on widening the nasal valve and providing support with cartilage grafts.

### Nonsurgical Management of Nasal Valve Collapse

For patients who are poor surgical candidates or hesitant about surgery, there are nonsurgical management options for nasal valve collapse. Various nasal strips act on the lateral wall to strengthen and relieve the propensity for nasal valve collapse by expanding the internal nasal valve. As an alternative, internal dilators can be commercially purchased, and when placed within the nasal passage, act to stent the airway.[3] There are a large variety of brands and devices but all act on either splinting the airway externally by providing support to the lateral wall and internal nasal valve, or internally by stenting the internal and external valves.

In addition, minimally invasive treatments have been developed for internal nasal valve collapse and to bolster lateral wall support. The Latera implant (Spirox Inc, Redwood City, CA, USA) can be placed in the office percutaneously through the vestibular skin on each side or the affected side of lateral wall collapse. The implant is made of an absorbable polymer material that will resorb over a period of approximately 18 months leaving a fibrous capsule in place that may provide additional support after the implant has dissolved.[5] Although the implant has only recently become available, preliminary clinical studies have shown improvement in nasal obstruction and reduction in NOSE scores.[6] Not only does the device have an impact on the internal nasal valve but also possibly on the external valve as well. The risks are minimal and include extrusion, minor bleeding, and low risk of infection.

The Latera device is initially marked with a positioning device and inserted endonasally stenting the internal valve and lateral wall (**Fig. 1**). It is important for the proximal aspect of the implant to remain above the alar crease with the distal aspect situated over the ipsilateral nasal bone. Local anesthesia is more than adequate for anesthesia during implantation and is highly effective. The implant is then loaded into the device and implanted into the previously marked plane taking care to insert above the alar crease and over the ipsilateral nasal bone (**Figs. 2** and **3**).

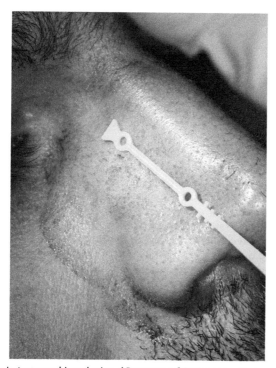

**Fig. 1.** The Spirox Latera marking device. (*Courtesy of* Spriox, Inc, Redwood City, CA.)

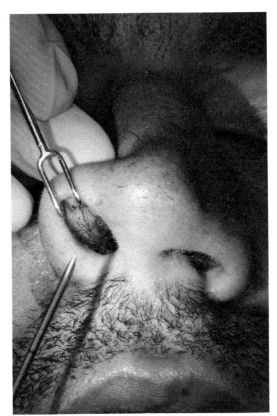

**Fig. 2.** Directed implantation of Latera above the supra-alar groove. (*Courtesy of* Spriox, Inc, Redwood City, CA.)

Although nonsurgical devices can be very successful in properly selected patients, surgical correction of nasal valve collapse is oftentimes required and various methods can lead to excellent results in functional and aesthetic rhinoplasty.

### Surgical Management of the Internal Nasal Valve

The internal nasal valve is one of the most frequently altered areas in performing septorhinoplasty. There are multiple surgical options available to open the internal nasal valve to improve breathing and also to alter the aesthetic appearance of the nose at the middle nasal vault. This can be accomplished by traditional spreader grafts, spreader flaps, butterfly grafts, and with additional support by batten grafts.[7] Regardless of the method, the goal is to expand the nasal valve area. The most commonly used method to improve obstruction at the internal nasal valve is spreader graft placement, although inferior turbinate reduction is becoming increasingly prominent, which is discussed later in this article.

Spreader grafts can be placed endonasally or via an external approach. They are placed submucosally under an intact connection between the upper lateral cartilage and dorsal septum to cantilever the upper lateral cartilage. Various autologous grafting materials can be used.

Spreader grafts are carved grafts, most commonly from septal cartilage, but in revision surgery or in extensive structural rhinoplasty, costal cartilage may be

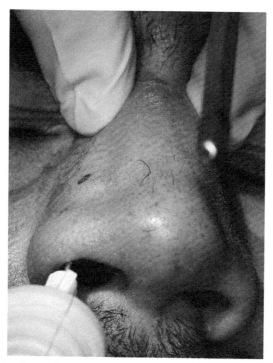

**Fig. 3.** Latera device inserted with palpation of the underlying nasal bone. (*Courtesy of Spriox, Inc, Redwood City, CA.*)

required (**Fig. 4**). The grafts are placed either into a submucosal pocket placed at the apex of the internal nasal valve, or between the upper lateral cartilage and dorsal septum after the soft tissue attachments between the 2 have been divided (**Figs. 5** and **6**). The length of the spreader grafts is dependent on the goals of reconstruction: sometimes the grafts need be extended underneath the nasal bones to provide support and maintain nasal bone position; other times the grafts need to be extended caudally for stabilization of a caudal septal extension graft. Because of the ability to alter length and width of the grafts, the spreader graft allows for the greatest versatility and is the preferred method of middle vault reconstruction.

Spreader flaps are less frequently used due to the thin nature of the upper lateral cartilage, but in certain patients can be appropriate. The spreader flap is crafted entirely from the upper lateral cartilage. Therefore, this cartilage needs to be strong but flexible. Initially, the upper lateral cartilage is released from the dorsal septum and the mucosa dissected from the undersurface of the upper lateral cartilage (**Fig. 7**). This is assisted by hydrodissection with 1% lidocaine with 1:100,000 epinephrine, which makes dissection in a subperichondrial plane easier. The medial aspect of the upper lateral cartilage is then folded on itself and sutured (**Fig. 8**). Oftentimes this requires a vertical incision at the apex of the flap that does not completely transect the upper lateral cartilage. Once the flap is sutured to itself, it is then secured to the dorsal septum (**Figs. 9** and **10**). Unfortunately, this technique is less versatile than the traditional spreader graft and allows for less control of the middle vault width. The cartilage here also tends to be more fragile and is more variable between patients, making the spreader flaps less predictable.

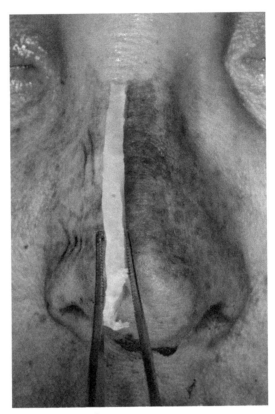

**Fig. 4.** Costal cartilage spreader graft.

Butterfly grafts, commonly harvested from the concha due to the natural curvature and flexibility of the cartilage, can also be used to stent open the internal nasal valve.[8] This graft was more frequently used in revision septorhinoplasty, although it has been described for use in the primary setting in patients with internal nasal valve collapse. Friedman and Cook[9] showed that patients undergoing primary septorhinoplasty with conchal cartilage butterfly graft, and had preexisting internal nasal valve collapse on modified Cottle maneuver, showed significant subjective improvement (90%) in nasal breathing.

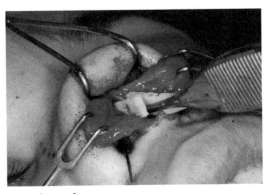

**Fig. 5.** Submucosal spreader graft.

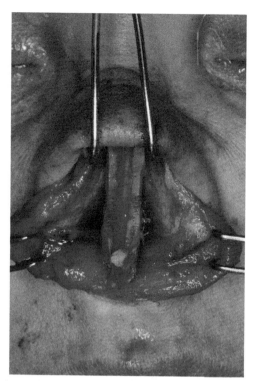

Fig. 6. Spreader grafts in place with a caudal septal extension graft.

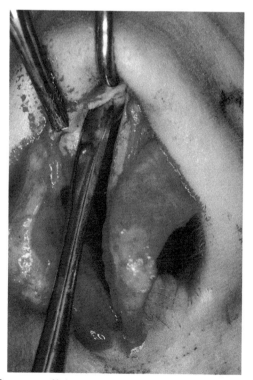

Fig. 7. Dissection of mucosa off the undersurface of the upper lateral cartilage.

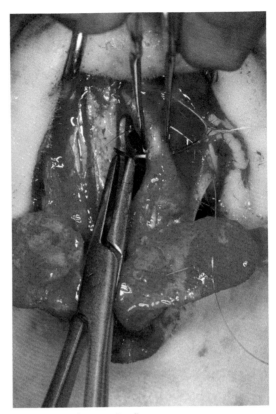

**Fig. 8.** Suture placement through spreader flap.

Finally, alar batten grafts can be used to bolster internal nasal valve support at the upper lateral cartilage. This technique is used in conjunction with spreader graft placement, which is useful in patients with severe lateral wall collapse. The batten graft is placed superficial to and sutured to the upper lateral cartilage.[10] The graft is easily placed and usually requires only a single suture to anchor the graft to the upper lateral cartilage. Batten grafts improve the strength and resistance of the upper lateral cartilage, which, in combination with other techniques, can improve patency of the internal nasal valve during inspiration. However, the authors think alar batten grafts are limited in their stability because they lack a medial support structure. The authors think the combination of lateral crural strut graft and obliquely angled dome sutures can effectively create a favorable tip contour in addition to improved support of the external nasal valve.

### Surgical Management of the External Valve/Lateral Wall

The lower lateral cartilages, composed of medial crus, intermediate crus, and lateral crus, play an important role in lateral wall support. The medial crus lies on either side of the caudal septum. Narrowing of the nostril can result from short or flared medial crura.[3] The shape and position of the lower lateral crus can contribute to external nasal valve obstruction. An internally concave lateral crus narrows the nasal vestibule and can lead to airway obstruction (**Figs. 11** and **12**). Cephalic malposition of the lower lateral cartilages is defined by the angle between the long axis of lateral crus as it moves away from the midline. An angle less than 28° to 30° is deemed

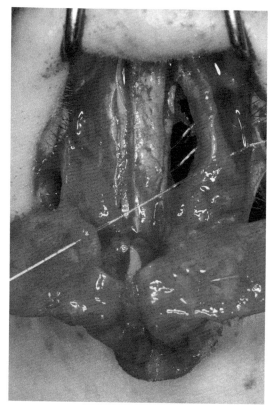

**Fig. 9.** Demonstration of a spreader graft before closure of the middle vault.

cephalically malpositioned. Of note, the lower lateral cartilages provide an archlike support to the nasal vestibule, supported medially by the septum and laterally by the lateral nasal sidewall. Lateral crural strut grafting provides a mechanism for correction of the lateral crura as it relates to nasal obstruction.[11]

A proper and precise understanding of lower lateral cartilage positioning has significant impact on nasal function and aesthetics. It is incumbent on the surgeon to recognize variant nasal anatomy. For example, failure to recognize cephalic positioning of the lateral crura can result in compromised nasal function because the lateral wall of the nose can collapse medially upon inspiration through the nose. Therefore, proper assessment of the cause of lateral wall weakness is critical to select proper grafting maneuvers, thus providing long-term aesthetic and functional outcomes.

Collapse of the lateral wall as it relates to nasal obstruction can be due to weakness of the lower lateral cartilage, cephalic malposition of the lower lateral cartilage, or concavity, all of which can be inherent to the patient anatomy or iatrogenic. Traditional reductive rhinoplasty with cephalic trim and dome sutures often leads to weakness of the lateral wall as well as concavity of the lateral crus, creating an unappealing aesthetic result and nasal valve obstruction. In the case of a concave or weak lateral crus that is caudally positioned, lateral crural strut grafts can be placed without repositioning to provide additional support to the lateral wall as well as flatten out the concavity of the lateral crus.[3] These grafts have the additional benefit of tip refinement and caudal rotation of the lateral crus.

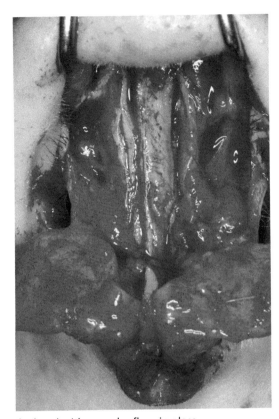

**Fig. 10.** Middle vault closed with spreader flaps in place.

Alternatively, in cephalically malpositioned lower lateral cartilages, repositioning is often required. Lateral crural repositioning begins with an open septorhinoplasty approach using hydrodissection with local anesthetic agent to assist in the dissection of the lateral crura from the underlying vestibular skin and eventual release of the crura from its most lateral attachments[11,12] (**Figs. 13** and **14**). Released lateral crura are repositioned into a more caudal orientation after suturing lateral crural strut grafts to the undersurface of the lateral crura (**Figs. 15–17**). Auricular cartilage is generally too weak, and septal cartilage is preferred. The lateral crural strut graft is fashioned with an angled medial edge, with the longer margin being placed just under the dome to move the caudal aspect of the dome anteriorly. A 5-0 PDS suture is used to secure the graft to the overlying lateral crura. Lateral crural repositioning can be further supplemented by domal sutures. The angle of the dome suture should be oriented so it is closer to the caudal margin medially and directed toward the cephalic margin laterally.[12] Then, creation of the lateral pocket for the placement of the lateral crural strut graft is made along the alar groove or just caudal to it. It is important to release the nasal envelope and assess for benefit in the repositioned cartilages. Furthermore, splinting of the nasal sidewall with clear plastic splints ensures the vestibular skin reattaches to the undersurface of the lateral crura and eliminates dead space that could add to thickness of the lateral wall.

Although proper management of the lateral wall and the apex of the internal nasal valve are essential for patency of the nasal airway, the septum and inferior turbinate also play a role in nasal valve obstruction.

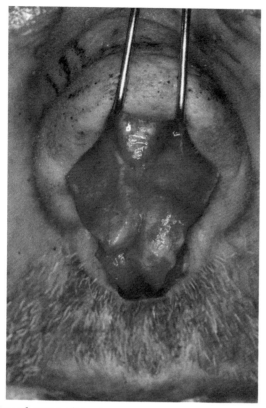

**Fig. 11.** Frontal view of concave lateral crura.

## Role of the Septum in Nasal Valve Obstruction

Management of the septum in regards to nasal valve collapse can be divided into management of the dorsal septum at the internal nasal valve and management of caudal septal deflections as they relate to nasal obstruction.

Dorsal septal deviations are most commonly seen in patients with a deviated nose and potential history of trauma. Vertical fractures through the dorsal strut can lead to significant destabilization of the lower third of the nose, while simultaneously causing obstruction at the internal nasal valve. The management of these deviations is primarily related to straightening of the dorsal septum with placement of spreader grafts, or asymmetrically placed middle vault sutures. In some cases, an asymmetrically placed middle vault suture can help correct a subtle tilt of the dorsal septum.[13] Other investigators have described the use of bow-tie sutures or mattress sutures, which can help straighten cartilage.[14]

Caudal septal deflections can be more complex depending on the degree of deviation and the relationship of the caudal septum to the anterior nasal spine (ANS), and the management is outside the scope of this article. If the caudal septum or ANS is off midline, the septum can be detached from the ANS and repositioned. This is accomplished by creating a small osteotomy at the ANS and repositioning the caudal septum, and anchoring with a 4-0 PDS suture. In severe deflections, extracorporeal septoplasty, or caudal septal replacement, often need to be used.

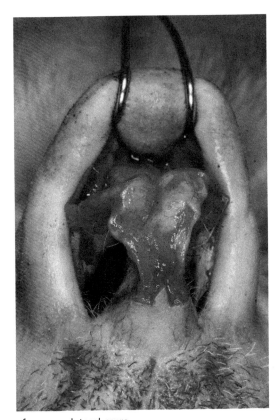

**Fig. 12.** Base view of concave lateral crura.

### Management of the Inferior Turbinate

The inferior turbinates can cause obstruction at the internal nasal valve due to compensatory hypertrophy primarily seen in combination with a deviated nasal septum. Inferior turbinates are incredibly important to normal nasal function, sensation of airflow and humidification of inhaled air. Conservative management of the inferior turbinate is strongly recommended because overreduction can lead to significant pathologic condition.

Surgical treatment of inferior turbinate hypertrophy is considered in symptomatic patients with turbinate hypertrophy and severe nasal obstruction who have failed medical management.[15] However, because of limited long-term follow-up studies, there is a lack of consensus for best surgical technique, timing, and patient selection for this surgical therapy. The surgical techniques used in inferior turbinate reduction are vast and include cryosurgery, thermal ablation, radiofrequency ablation, powered instrument reduction, ultrasound reduction, submucosal resection, or turbinectomy (partial or total). The authors advocate highly for mucosal-sparing techniques as atrophic rhinitis, or empty nose syndrome, is a potential sequelae of overreduction of the inferior turbinate, especially with ablative or thermal techniques that cause significant damage to the mucosa. This frequently causes significant dryness, feeling of suffocation within the nose, and pain that leads to some patients to becoming depressed or even suicidal.

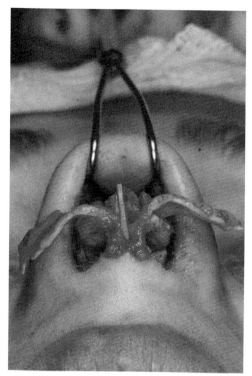

**Fig. 13.** Base view of released lateral crura.

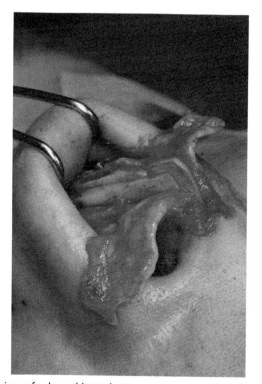

**Fig. 14.** Surgeon's view of released lateral crura.

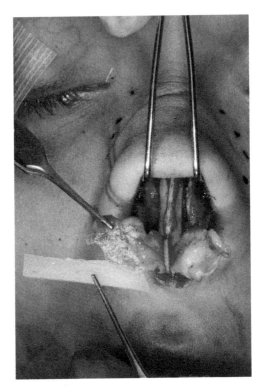

**Fig. 15.** Lateral crural strut graft.

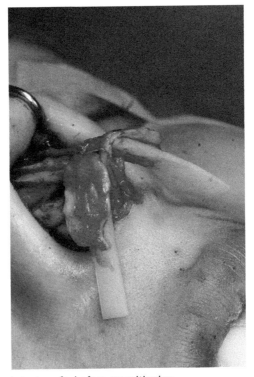

**Fig. 16.** Lateral crural strut grafts before repositioning.

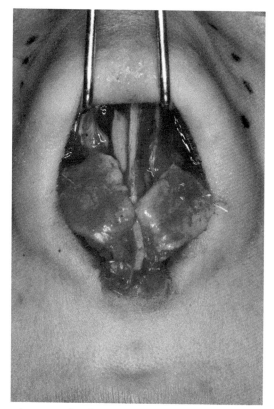

**Fig. 17.** Lateral crural strut grafts after repositioning maneuver.

## SUMMARY

In summary, nasal valve collapse is a well-known entity with a complex array of treatment options ranging from nonsurgical splints to surgical nasal reconstruction with extensive grafting. Each case presents its own unique variation, and patients must be addressed individually, targeting the areas of weakness that can be corrected.

## REFERENCES

1. Khosh MM, Jen A, Honrad C, et al. Nasal valve reconstruction: experience in 53 consecutive patients. Arch Facial Plast Surg 2004;6(3):167–71.
2. Constantian M. Differing characteristics in 100 consecutive secondary rhinoplasty patients following closed versus open surgical approaches. Plast Reconstr Surg 2002;109(6):2097–111.
3. Hamilton GS II. The external nasal valve. Facial Plast Surg Clin North Am 2017;25: 179–94.
4. Stewart MG, Witsell DL, Smith TL, et al. Development and validation of the nasal obstruction symptom evaluation (NOSE) scale. Otolaryngol Head Neck Surg 2004;130(2):157–63.
5. Spirox latera™ implant support of lateral nasal wall cartilage (LATERAL-OR) study. Spirox; 2016.

6. San Nicolo M, Stelter K, Sadick H, et al. Absorbable implant to treat nasal valve collapse. Facial Plast Surg 2017;33(2):233–40.
7. Rhee JS, Arganbright JM, Mcmullin BT, et al. Evidence supporting functional rhinoplasty or nasal valve repair: a 25-year systematic review. Otolaryngol Head Neck Surg 2008;139(1):10–20.
8. Clark JM, Cook TA. The 'Butterfly' graft in functional secondary rhinoplasty. Laryngoscope 2002;112(11):1917–25.
9. Friedman O, Cook TA. Conchal cartilage butterfly graft in primary functional rhinoplasty. Laryngoscope 2009;119(2):255–62.
10. Toriumi DM, Josen J, Weinberger M, et al. Use of alar batten grafts for correction of nasal valve collapse. Arch Otolaryngol Head Neck Surg 1997;123:802–8.
11. Gunter JP, Friedman RM. Lateral crural strut graft. Technique and clinical applications in rhinoplasty. Plast Reconstr Surg 1997;109:943–55.
12. Toriumi DM, Asher SA. Lateral crural repositioning for treatment of cephalic malposition. Facial Plast Surg Clin North Am 2015;23(1):55–71.
13. Moubayed SP, Most SP. Correction deviations of the lower 1/3rd of the nose. Facial Plast Surg 2017;33(2):157–61.
14. Miller PJ, Dayan SH. The bow-tie mattress suture for correction of nasal cartilage convexities and concavities. Arch Facial Plast Surg 2010;12(5):354–6.
15. Fraser L, Kelly G. An evidence-based approach to the management of the adult with nasal obstruction. Clin Otolaryngol 2009;34(2):151–5.

# Surgical Management of Nonallergic Rhinitis

Carol H. Yan, MD, Peter H. Hwang, MD*

## KEYWORDS

- Nonallergic rhinitis • Vasomotor rhinitis • Nasal congestion • Rhinorrhea
- Vidian neurectomy • Posterior nasal neurectomy • Cryotherapy

## KEY POINTS

- Vasomotor rhinitis is the most frequent subtype of nonallergic rhinitis (NAR) and is characterized by non–immunoglobulin E–mediated symptoms of nasal congestion, obstruction, and rhinorrhea.
- NAR is triggered by changes in environmental conditions, weather, strong emotions, smells, and hormones.
- Although medical management is the first-line treatment of NAR, there is a role for surgical therapy when medications fail to improve symptoms.
- Vasomotor rhinitis is due, in part, to an imbalance between parasympathetic and sympathetic inputs to the autonomic nervous system.
- Surgical targeting of the vidian nerve and its branches can result in symptomatic improvement. Options include vidian neurectomy, posterior nasal neurectomy, and cryotherapy.

## INTRODUCTION

Nonallergic rhinitis (NAR) describes chronic symptoms of nasal congestion, obstruction, and rhinorrhea unrelated to a specific allergen based on skin or serum testing. NAR affects approximately 30 million Americans, and more than 200 million worldwide.[1] Although NAR can present with symptoms similar to those found in allergic rhinitis (AR), NAR tends to have an older age of onset, typically presenting between 30 and 60 years of life.[2] Patients with NAR are more commonly women, have decreased eosinophil response, and suffer from more frequent headaches and olfactory dysfunction, but less sneezing and pruritus.[3] The predominant symptom of NAR, nasal congestion, can have a significant impact on quality of life, contributing to sleep disturbances, daytime somnolence, and decreased productivity at work. Additionally, patients may have a combination of AR and NAR, known as mixed rhinitis (MR). The

Disclosure Statement: P.H. Hwang- Consultant for Arrinex, Inc. C.H. Yan has nothing to disclose.
Department of Otolaryngology–Head and Neck Surgery, Stanford University School of Medicine, 801 Welch Road, Stanford, CA 94305, USA
* Corresponding author.
E-mail address: hwangph@stanford.edu

Otolaryngol Clin N Am 51 (2018) 945–955
https://doi.org/10.1016/j.otc.2018.05.010
oto.theclinics.com

use of an irritant index questionnaire has helped to reclassify patients with NAR, AR, or MR based on their symptoms in response to nonallergic triggers and aeroallergen skin prick tests, as well as to stratify them according to low or high irritant burdens.[4] Patients with NAR are often misdiagnosed as having sinusitis and are treated with multiple courses of antibiotics without resolution of symptoms.

In recent years, NAR has been divided into several different subtypes, including rhinitis that is drug-induced, gustatory, hormonal, or senile; vasomotor rhinitis (VMR); NAR with eosinophilia; and atrophic rhinitis.[5] VMR is the most frequent form of NAR and is characterized by nasal symptoms usually triggered by changes in environmental conditions, weather, strong emotions, smells, and hormones. Brandt and Bernstein[6] developed a validated questionnaire that helps diagnose VMR. Unlike AR, VMR is a clinical diagnosis based on a patient's symptoms and triggers.

To best appreciate the treatment options for NAR, we need to first evaluate the pathophysiology of NAR. Although the etiology is not well understood, there is thought to be a dysregulation of sympathetic, parasympathetic, and nociceptive nerves innervating the nasal mucosa resulting in increased vascular permeability and mucus release from submucosal nasal glands.[7,8] Mucus secretion is controlled primarily by the parasympathetic nervous system, whereas the sympathetic system controls the vascular tone.[9] Acetylcholine is the main parasympathetic neurotransmitter that regulates nasal mucus secretion and rhinorrhea, a common symptom of rhinitis. Noradrenaline and neuropeptide Y are sympathetic neurotransmitters that modulate the secretions initiated by the parasympathetic system.[10] In addition, sensory neuropeptides and nociceptive type C-fibers of the trigeminal nerve contribute to mast cell degranulation and the itching and sneezing reflexes.

The first-line treatment for VMR is medical therapy in the form of topical corticosteroid and topical antihistamine sprays (which are indicated for NAR as well as AR). Ipratropium bromide (0.03%) is the only topical anticholinergic approved for treatment of NAR with no systemic side effects except for occasional dryness and epistaxis.[11] Topical capsaicin has been shown to be an efficacious treatment for NAR based on its modulating effects on C-fibers, but because of its irritant qualities, its use is often limited by patient intolerance.[12] There are no oral antihistamines or anticholinergics currently approved for NAR. When medical management does not adequately control a patient's symptoms, surgical interventions may be considered (**Fig. 1**).

## INFERIOR TURBINATE REDUCTION

Inferior turbinate hypertrophy contributes to chronic rhinitis symptomatology by hypersecretion and nasal obstruction. Patients with NAR have been shown to benefit from surgical corrections of nasal obstruction with improvements in the patient-reported sino-nasal outcome test (SNOT-22), global nasal function tests, and objective nasal peak inspiratory flow.[13]

Many different surgical techniques have been developed for inferior turbinate reduction (ITR). The total inferior turbinectomy, historically performed to improve nasal obstruction, has long fallen out of favor, as it can lead to potential complications, including atrophic rhinitis and paradoxic nasal obstruction, characteristic of empty nose syndrome.[14] Mucosal-sparing and turbinate-sparing techniques are now favored to preserve physiologic function of the turbinate; they include submucosal microdebrider reduction of soft tissue, submucosal resection of bone, electrocautery, radiofrequency ablation, coblation, laser ablation, cryotherapy, direct microdebridement, and

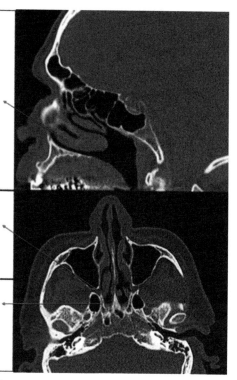

**Inferior Turbinate**
- Submucous Turbinate Reduction (soft tissue ± bone)
- Electrocautery Ablation
- Radiofrequency Ablation
- Coblation
- Laser Ablation
- Microdebridement
- Lateral Bone Outfracture
- Botulinum Toxin

**Posterior Nerve**
- Posterior Nerve Neurectomy
- Posterior Nerve Cryoabalation

**Vidian Nerve**
- Vidian Neurectomy
  - Endoscopic Antegrade approach
  - Endoscopic Retrograde approach

**Fig. 1.** Surgical targets in vasomotor rhinitis.

lateral bone outfracture. The pros and cons of each technique are well studied and described. In general, there is abundant level 3 and 4 evidence supporting the benefit of various modalities of turbinate reduction in patients with VMR.[15–19] However, no true standard of care exists because robust side-by-side comparisons of turbinate reduction techniques have not been done.

In one study attempting such a comparison, Passali and colleagues[20] performed one of the few randomized control trials evaluating 6 surgical techniques for inferior turbinate reduction with a 6-year follow-up period. The investigators compared traditional turbinate resection, laser cautery, electrocautery, cryotherapy, submucosal resection, and submucosal resection with lateral bone displacement. Of the 6 options, only submucosal resection resulted in stable subjective symptom improvement in nasal obstruction and discharge as well as objective improved mucociliary clearance and nasal volumes. The addition of lateral bony displacement further improved long-term results. More recently, Harju and colleagues[21] conducted a randomized placebo-controlled trial of turbinate reduction techniques, comparing radiofrequency ablation, diode laser, and microdebrider-assisted inferior turbinoplasty, as well as a sham procedure. Although the sham procedure was associated with a notable placebo effect of patient-reported improvement, all 3 surgical techniques provided statistically significant additional reductions in severity of nasal obstruction compared with the sham procedure. There was no superior technique among the 3 tested. Regardless of the technique, the overarching goal in inferior turbinate surgery remains to improve the nasal airway and decrease mucosal edema while preserving turbinate function.

## BOTULINUM TOXIN

Botulinum toxin (BTX) has been shown to have a potential role in treatment of NAR through its anticholinergic effect on nasal mucosa.[9] BTX inhibits the release of acetylcholine from the presynaptic nerve terminal; of the available serotypes, BTX-A has the greatest anticholinergic effect. The injection of BTX-A (4 U) into the head of the inferior (2 U) and middle turbinates (2 U) in patients with VMR decreases rhinorrhea, but the improvement is typically short-lived, lasting only 4 weeks.[22] Injection of higher doses of BTX-A (20 U) decreases symptoms of nasal obstruction, sneezing, nasal discharge, and nasal itching for up to 12 weeks.[23] BTX also can be safely injected into the septum at higher doses (80 U), but the improvement in nasal symptoms is short-lived at only 2 weeks.[24] All studies have shown BTX injection to be safe and without significant side effects. However, BTX may not be a practical option for most patients with VMR, given that the symptom benefits are only temporary. In addition, only the rhinorrhea symptom of VMR is reduced by BTX. Furthermore, not all patients see an improvement with BTX, likely due to the multifactorial causes of rhinitis that are not mediated by acetylcholine.[25]

## VIDIAN NEURECTOMY

Therapeutic transection of the vidian nerve is a well-described surgical option that aims to disrupt the autonomic supply to the nasal cavity, thereby decreasing nasal secretions. The vidian nerve is formed by the joining of the greater superficial petrosal and deep petrosal nerves. The deep petrosal nerve contains sympathetic fibers, whereas the greater superficial petrosal nerve contains preganglionic parasympathetic secretomotor fibers for the lacrimal, palatine, and nasal glands, as well as the vasodilator nerves for the nasal mucous membranes.[26] The first vidian neurectomy was described by Golding-Wood[27] in 1961 through a transantral approach. Others described performing neurectomies using transpalatal, transethmoidal, and transnasal techniques.[28] However, these initial surgeries suffered from significant morbidity due to postoperative bleeding, facial and palate numbness, and ocular injuries.[29] Recurrent symptoms from incomplete nerve section was common due to poor visualization afforded by these approaches. The popularity of the vidian neurectomy diminished until the application of endoscopic techniques, which have improved visualization and decreased complications.

El Shazly[30] in 1991 described one of the earliest reports of endoscopic vidian neurectomy with successful resolution of secretomotor rhinitis symptoms. Robinson and Wormald[26] subsequently described their retrograde endoscopic technique by which a mucosal incision is made over the sphenopalatine foramen and the sphenopalatine artery is cauterized. A mucosal flap is elevated posteriorly to the anterior face of the sphenoid and the periosteum and fat of the pterygopalatine fossa is exposed. The vidian nerve, which travels along the sphenoid floor, is identified emerging through the pterygoid canal (**Fig. 2**). The nerve is isolated and sharply resected and cauterized. Another technique proposed by Su and colleagues[31] uses an anterograde transsphenoidal approach to the vidian nerve by first creating a large sphenoidotomy and removing the sphenoid process of the palatine bone until the vidian canal is identified inferolaterally. This anterograde approach obviates the need to ligate the sphenopalatine artery. Both techniques recommend resection of a 2-mm to 3-mm segment of the vidian nerve in addition to cautery of the nerve stump to prevent reinnervation.

Endoscopic vidian neurectomy has benefited from an improvement in intraoperative visualization, yielding increased success rates. Rates of successful control of rhinitis and of patient satisfaction have been reported as high as 91% after vidian

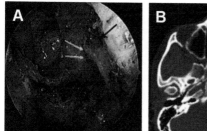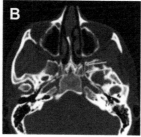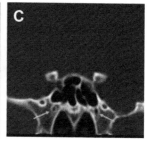

**Fig. 2.** (*A*) Endoscopic view of the vidian canal drilled along its medial and inferior borders (*blue arrows*), beginning at its opening in the posterior pterygopalatine fossa (*black arrow*). Axial (*B*) and coronal (*C*) computed tomography views of the vidian canal (*blue arrows*) at the base of the sphenoid sinus. (*From* [A] Oakley GM, Harvey RJ. Endoscopic resection of pterygopalatine fossa and infratemporal fossa malignancies. Otolaryngol Clin North Am 2017;50:2; with permission.)

neurectomy.[32,33] A recent systematic review by Marshak and colleagues[34] reported that all published case series that used the endoscopic technique for VMR had an improvement in rhinorrhea and nasal obstruction. In one of the only prospective case series published, Zhang and colleagues[35] showed improvement in patients' reported Sinusitis Symptom Questionnaire scores and SNOT-22 scores, particularly in the subdomains of rhinorrhea and nasal congestion.

Despite favorable success rates with vidian neurectomy, there can be notable complications associated with the procedure. The most commonly cited complication is postoperative dry eyes due to collateral injury of the postganglionic secretomotory fibers innervating the lacrimal gland. Halderman and Sindwani[29] systematically reviewed 6 studies that described endoscopic vidian neurectomies. The rate of dry eyes ranged from 23.8% to 100.0% with an aggregate rate of 48.0%. The second most common complication was cheek, palate, and gingival numbness that ranged from 2.97% to 22.2% in reviewed studies.[29] However, most of the symptoms were temporary, with dry eyes resolving in 1 to 6 months and cheek/palate numbness resolving between 2 weeks and 1 year.[34]

## POSTERIOR NASAL NEURECTOMY

In light of concerns regarding complications that may be associated with vidian neurectomy, the posterior nasal nerve has emerged as an alternative surgical target. The vidian nerve travels through the pterygoid canal as a single bundle until its parasympathetic fibers synapse at the sphenopalatine ganglion. The postganglionic fibers consist of multiple efferent rami that project from the pterygopalatine ganglion to separately innervate the orbit, palate, and nasal mucosa.[36] The postsynaptic parasympathetic fibers that give rise to the posterior nasal nerve travel with the sphenopalatine artery, entering the nasal cavity via the sphenopalatine foramen. Because the posterior nasal nerve traverses distal to the branching point for nerves innervating the lacrimal gland and palate, selective transnasal sectioning of the posterior nasal nerve does not carry a risk of eye dryness or palate numbness. In rat models, transection of the posterior nasal nerve results in depletion of choline acetyltransferase and a twofold reduction in nasal secretions.[37]

Kikawada[38] first described the posterior nasal neurectomy (PNN) as an alternative to vidian neurectomy (**Fig. 3**). A vertical incision is made in the posterior middle meatus

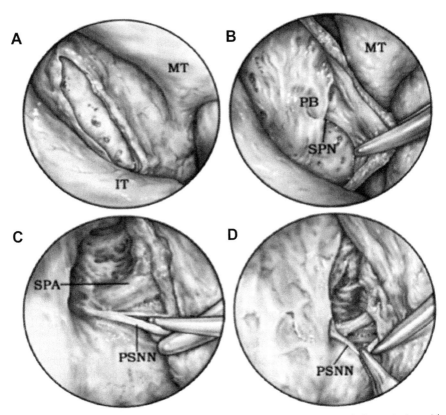

**Fig. 3.** Endoscopic posterior nerve neurectomy (*A*). Vertical incision made in posterior middle meatus (*B*). Sphenopalatine palatine bundle identified at sphenopalatine notch (*C*, *D*). Posterior superior nasal nerves separated from sphenopalatine artery and ligated. IT, inferior turbinate; MT, middle turbinate; PB, palatine bone; PSNN, posterior superior nasal nerve; SPA, sphenopalatine artery; SPN, sphenopalatine notch. (*Adapted from* Kikawada T. Endoscopic posterior nasal neurectomy: an alternative to vidian neurectomy. Oper Tech Otolayngol Head Neck Surg 2007;18:4; with permission.)

over the perpendicular process of the palatine bone, a mucoperiosteal flap is elevated over the palatine bone, and the sphenopalatine foramen (SPF) can be identified immediately posterior to the crista ethmoidalis. The posterior nasal nerve can be identified emerging from the SPF, within the neurovascular bundle containing the nerve and the sphenopalatine vessels. The entire sphenopalatine bundle (nerve and artery) can be ligated together when performing the PNN, or the nerve and its branches can be dissected free from the artery and transected separately (**Fig. 4**).[39] Alternatively, a transturbinate approach has been described. From an anterior incision in the inferior turbinate, a submucoperiosteal dissection is performed until the SPF is identified. The neural bundle can be visualized exiting the SPF toward the inferior turbinate.[40] After PNN has been performed, a submucosal resection of the inferior turbinate soft tissue can be performed through the same incision.[41]

The efficacy of the PNN procedure has not been studied as thoroughly as that of vidian neurectomy. There is currently a paucity of literature that evaluates the outcomes of PNN for NAR specifically. Two recent systematic reviews performed found

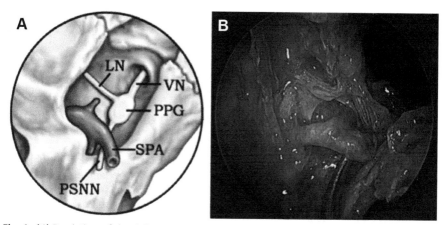

**Fig. 4.** (A) Depiction of the right posterior superior nasal nerve (PSNN) and vidian nerve (VN) and their relationship to the sphenopalatine artery (SPA). (B) Isolation of the SPA as it passes through the sphenopalatine foramen. LN, lacrimal nerve; PPG, pterygopalatine ganglion. (*Adapted from* [A] Kikawada T. Endoscopic posterior nasal neurectomy: an alternative to vidian neurectomy. Oper Tech Otolayngol Head Neck Surg 2007;18:4; with permission.)

that most studies discussed the effects of PNN on patients with AR.[29,34] As the only outcomes study that included patients with NAR, Ikeda and colleagues[41] performed 56 PNN procedures in patients with recalcitrant AR or NAR and noted a $\geq$80% improvement in total symptomatic scores for 86% of the patients. In patients with AR, Kobayashi and colleagues[40] reported significant improvement in sneezing, rhinorrhea, and nasal obstruction after transturbinate neurectomy of peripheral branches of the posterior nasal nerve; the addition of a concurrently performed transection of the main posterior nasal nerve did not result in further improvement. In human histologic studies, the post-PNN nasal cavity demonstrates decreases in the density of nasal gland cells and inflammatory cells.[42] Cassano and colleagues[43] noted improved mucociliary transport time in patients with VMR who underwent sphenopalatine artery ligation and PNN with ITR compared with those who underwent ITR alone.

Despite the symptomatic improvements and low complication rate associated with PNN, some patients may not have a complete response after PNN. This may be because of gradual postoperative reinnervation,[37] or to the presence of persistent accessory secretomotor fibers to the posterolateral mucosa that do not transverse the sphenopalatine foramen.[44] In 90% of cadaver models studied, additional rami were found traversing the perpendicular process of the palatine bone that were separate from the contributions found in the sphenopalatine foramen. Histologic studies confirmed the presence of these autonomic fibers.[45] Thus, to perform a complete postganglionic pterygopalatine parasympathectomy, one must meticulously trace and transect the array of these accessory fibers in addition to the primary posterior nasal nerve to fully denervate the nasal mucosa.[45]

## CRYOABLATION OF THE POSTERIOR NASAL NERVE

Cryotherapy has been safely used in the head and neck region for soft tissue ablation for several indications. Cryotherapy offers unique advantages to other forms of tissue ablation in that the zone of injury is predictably superficial, allowing for the ablation of nerve while preserving the patency of the associated vasculature. The use of cryosurgical therapy for rhinitis was first proposed in 1970 with the placement of a cryoprobe in the nasal cavity against the posterior end of the inferior turbinate.[46] The procedure showed promising efficacy; however, the investigators reported complications of serous otitis media and septal perforations. These complications were likely related to imprecise application of cryogen, perhaps exacerbated by poor visualization of the posterior nasal cavity without the benefit of endoscopic visualization. The requirement for very large cryogen reservoirs and nonergonomic cryoprobes also contributed to the limited adoption of cryotherapy technology at the time.

Recently, cryotherapy has reemerged as a modality for ablating the posterior nasal nerve in an office-based setting, obviating the need for general anesthesia. Interest in cryoablative technology was revived with the introduction of an in-office cryosurgical ablation device developed to deliver cryogen to the posterior middle meatus and freeze the posterior nasal nerve under endoscopic visualization (Arrinex Inc, Redwood City, CA) (**Fig. 5**).[47] A study of office-based cryotherapy in patients with VMR and AR demonstrated that patients' Total Nasal Symptom Score decreased significantly up to 365 days after treatment, particularly in the symptoms of rhinorrhea and congestion.[47] There were no postoperative instances of dry eyes or palate numbness.

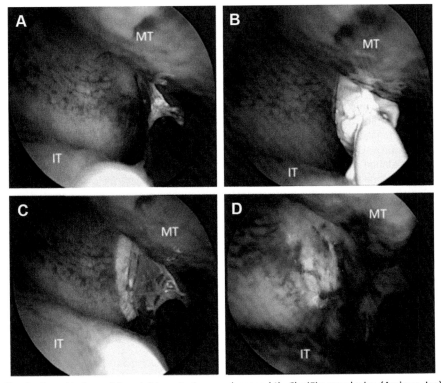

**Fig. 5.** Cryoablation of the right posterior nasal nerve (A). ClariFix cryodevice (Arrinex, Inc) placed endoscopically in posterior middle meatus (B). Activation of cryogen (C, D). Evidence of cryoablation with tissue blanching on withdrawal of the cryodevice. IT, inferior turbinate; MT, middle turbinate. (Courtesy of Arrinex, Inc, Redwood City, CA.)

## KINETIC OSCILLATION STIMULATION

Kinetic oscillation stimulation (KOS) is an application of low-frequency, low-amplitude mechanical oscillations to simulate turbulent nasal airflow in an effort to reduce inflammatory response in the nose. A preliminary study suggested the use of a KOS device improved the nasal symptoms of obstruction, itchiness, and secretion for up to 2 weeks compared with a placebo.[48] However, little is known currently about this device's mechanism of action. A second randomized clinical trial using KOS for treatment of NAR is under way (clinical trials.gov: NCT03399721).

## SUMMARY

NAR, including vasomotor rhinitis, is a common disease that impairs the quality of life of many patients. Medical therapy is first-line treatment, but when treatments do not provide adequate relief, there is a role for surgical management. Turbinate reduction surgery yields well-studied benefits. More directed targeting of the underlying autonomic dysfunction in NAR through endoscopic vidian neurectomy and PNN have been shown to be effective in reducing symptoms of chronic rhinitis, particularly congestion and rhinorrhea. The PNN has far lower rates of dry eye complications although its efficacy is not as well established. The desire for in-office treatment options makes botulinum toxin injection and cryotherapy of the posterior nasal nerve potentially attractive options, but larger studies are required to characterize their long-term treatment effects.

## REFERENCES

1. Scarupa MD, Kaliner MA. Nonallergic rhinitis, with a focus on vasomotor rhinitis: clinical importance, differential diagnosis, and effective treatment recommendations. World Allergy Organ J 2009;2:20–5.
2. Settipane RA, Charnock DR. Epidemiology of rhinitis: allergic and nonallergic. Clin Allergy Immunol 2007;19:23–34.
3. Di Lorenzo G, Pacor ML, Amodio E, et al. Differences and similarities between allergic and nonallergic rhinitis in a large sample of adult patients with rhinitis symptoms. Int Arch Allergy Immunol 2011;155:263–70.
4. Bernstein JA, Levin LS, Al-Shuik E, et al. Clinical characteristics of chronic rhinitis patients with high vs low irritant trigger burdens. Ann Allergy Asthma Immunol 2012;109:173–8.
5. Kaliner MA. Classification of nonallergic rhinitis syndromes with a focus on vasomotor rhinitis, proposed to be known henceforth as nonallergic rhinopathy. World Allergy Organ J 2009;2:98–101.
6. Brandt D, Bernstein JA. Questionnaire evaluation and risk factor identification for nonallergic vasomotor rhinitis. Ann Allergy Asthma Immunol 2006;96(4):526–32.
7. Bernstein JA. Nonallergic rhinitis: therapeutic options. Curr Opin Allergy Clin Immunol 2013;13:410–6.
8. Joe SA. Nonallergic rhinitis. Facial Plast Surg Clin North Am 2012;20:21–30.
9. Shaari CM, Sanders I, Wu BL, et al. Rhinorrhea is decreased in dogs after nasal application of botulinum toxin. Otolaryngol Head Neck Surg 1995;112(4):566–71.
10. Ozcan C, Ismi O. Botulinum toxin for rhinitis. Curr Allergy Asthma Rep 2016;16(8):58.
11. Bronsky EA, Druce H, Findlay SR, et al. A clinical trial of ipratropium bromide nasal spray in patients with perennial nonallergic rhinitis. J Allergy Clin Immunol 1995;95(5 Pt 2):1117–22.

12. Gevorgyan A, Segboer C, Gorissen R, et al. Capsaicin for non-allergic rhinitis. Cochrane Database Syst Rev 2015;(7):CD010591.
13. Parthasarathi K, Christensen JM, Alvarado R, et al. Airflow and symptom outcomes between allergic and non-allergic rhinitis patients from turbinoplasty. Rhinology 2017;55(4):332–8.
14. Moore GF, Freeman TJ, Ogren FP, et al. Extended follow-up of total inferior turbinate resection for relief of chronic nasal obstruction. Laryngoscope 1985;95(9 Pt 1):1095–9.
15. Deenadayal DS, Kumar MN, Sudhakshin P, et al. Radiofrequency reduction of inferior turbinates in allergic and non allergic rhinitis. Indian J Otolaryngol Head Neck Surg 2014;66(Suppl 1):231–6.
16. Bhattacharyya N, Kepnes LJ. Clinical effectiveness of coblation inferior turbinate reduction. Otolaryngol Head Neck Surg 2003;129(4):365–71.
17. Assanasen P, Banhiran W, Tantilipikorn P, et al. Combined radiofrequency volumetric tissue reduction and lateral outfracture of hypertrophic inferior turbinate in the treatment of chronic rhinitis: short-term and long-term outcome. Int Forum Allergy Rhinol 2014;4(4):339–44.
18. Sroka R, Janda P, Killian T, et al. Comparison of long term results after Ho:YAG and diode laser treatment of hyperplastic inferior nasal turbinates. Lasers Surg Med 2007;39(4):324–31.
19. Bouetel V, Lescanne E, Bakhos D, et al. Microdebrider-assisted partial turbinoplasty: technique and results in perennial non-allergic rhinitis. Rev Laryngol Otol Rhinol (Bord) 2009;130(4–5):261–6 [in French].
20. Passali D, Passali FM, Damiani V, et al. Treatment of inferior turbinate hypertrophy: a randomized clinical trial. Ann Otol Rhinol Laryngol 2003;112(8):683–8.
21. Harju T, Numminen J, Kivekas I, et al. A prospective, randomized, placebo-controlled study of inferior turbinate surgery. Laryngoscope 2018. https://doi.org/10.1002/lary.27103.
22. Kim KS, Kim SS, Yoon JH, et al. The effect of botulinum toxin type A injection for intrinsic rhinitis. J Laryngol Otol 1998;112(3):248–51.
23. Ozcan C, Vayisoglu Y, Dogu O, et al. The effect of intranasal injection of botulinum toxin A on the symptoms of vasomotor rhinitis. Am J Otolaryngol 2006;27(5):314–8.
24. Braun T, Gurkov R, Kramer MF, et al. Septal injection of botulinum neurotoxin A for idiopathic rhinitis: a pilot study. Am J Otolaryngol 2012;33(1):64–7.
25. Rohrbach S, Junghans K, Kohler S, et al. Minimally invasive application of botulinum toxin A in patients with idiopathic rhinitis. Head Face Med 2009;5:18.
26. Robinson SR, Wormald PJ. Endoscopic vidian neurectomy. Am J Rhinol 2006;20(2):197–202.
27. Golding-Wood PH. Observations on petrosal and vidian neurectomy in chronic vasomotor rhinitis. J Laryngol Otol 1961;75:232–47.
28. Osawa S, Rhoton AL, Seker A, et al. Microsurgical and endoscopic anatomy of the vidian canal. Neurosurgery 2009;64:385–411 [discussion: 411–2].
29. Halderman A, Sindwani R. Surgical management of vasomotor rhinitis: a systematic review. Am J Rhinol Allergy 2015;29:128–34.
30. el Shazly MA. Endoscopic surgery of the vidian nerve. Preliminary report. Ann Otol Rhinol Laryngol 1991;100(7):536–9.
31. Su WF, Liu SC, Chiu FS, et al. Antegrade transsphenoidal vidian neurectomy: short-term surgical outcome analysis. Am J Rhinol Allergy 2011;25(6):e217–20.
32. Ma Y, Tan G, Zhao Z, et al. Therapeutic effectiveness of endoscopic vidian neurectomy for the treatment of vasomotor rhinitis. Acta Otolaryngol 2014;134:260–7.

33. Lee JC, Kao CH, Hsu CH, et al. Endoscopic transsphenoidal vidian neurectomy. Eur Arch Otorhinolaryngol 2011;268(6):851–6.
34. Marshak T, Yun WK, Hazout C, et al. A systematic review of the evidence base for vidian neurectomy in managing rhinitis. J Laryngol Otol 2016;130(Suppl 4): S7–28.
35. Zhang H, Micomonaco DC, Dziegielewski PT, et al. Endoscopic vidian neurectomy: a prospective case series. Int Forum Allergy Rhinol 2015;5:423–30.
36. Ruskell GL. Orbital passage of pterygopalatine ganglion efferents to paranasal sinuses and nasal mucosa in man. Cells Tissues Organs 2003;175(4):223–8.
37. Nishijima H, Kondo K, Toma-Hirano M, et al. Prolonged denervation induces remodeling of nasal mucosa in rat model of posterior nasal neurectomy. Int Forum Allergy Rhinol 2017;7(7):670–8.
38. Kikawada T. Endoscopic posterior nasal neurectomy: an alternative to vidian neurectomy. Oper Tech Otolayngol Head Neck Surg 2007;18(4):297–301.
39. Eren E, Zeybek G, Ecevit C, et al. A new method of identifying the posterior inferior nasal nerve: implications for posterior nasal neurectomy. J Craniofac Surg 2015;26(3):930–2.
40. Kobayashi T, Hyodo M, Nakamura K, et al. Resection of peripheral branches of the posterior nasal nerve compared to conventional posterior neurectomy in severe allergic rhinitis. Auris Nasus Larynx 2012;39:593–6.
41. Ikeda K, Oshima T, Suzuki M, et al. Functional inferior turbinosurgery (FITS) for the treatment of resistant chronic rhinitis. Acta Otolaryngol 2006;126(7):739–45.
42. Ikeda K, Yokoi H, Saito T, et al. Effect of resection of the posterior nasal nerve on functional and morphological changes in the inferior turbinate mucosa. Acta Otolaryngol 2008;128(12):1337–41.
43. Cassano M, Russo L, Del Giudice AM, et al. Cytologic alterations in nasal mucosa after sphenopalatine artery ligation in patients with vasomotor rhinitis. Am J Rhinol Allergy 2012;26:49–54.
44. Bleier BS, Schlosser RJ. Endoscopic anatomy of the postganglionic pterygopalatine innervation of the posterolateral nasal mucosa. Int Forum Allergy Rhinol 2011;1(2):113–7.
45. Bleier BS, Feldman R, Sadow PM, et al. The accessory posterolateral nerve: an immunohistological analysis. Am J Rhinol Allergy 2012;26(4):271–3.
46. Ozenberger JM. Cryosurgery in chronic rhinitis. Laryngoscope 1970;80(5): 723–34.
47. Hwang PH, Lin B, Weiss R, et al. Cryosurgical posterior nasal tissue ablation for the treatment of rhinitis. Int Forum Allergy Rhinol 2017;7(10):952–6.
48. Juto JE, Axelsson M. Kinetic oscillation stimulation as treatment of non-allergic rhinitis: an RCT study. Acta Otolaryngol 2014;134(5):506–12.

# Office-Based Procedures for Nasal Airway Obstruction

Nadim Bikhazi, MD[a], James H. Atkins, MD[b],*

## KEYWORDS

- Office procedures • In-office • Septoplasty • Nasal valve repair • Turbinate surgery
- Septoplasty

## KEY POINTS

- The frequency of office procedures for nasal obstruction has increased in response to patient preference and payer patterns.
- The most common in-office procedures are turbinate surgery, nasal valve repair with Latera, posterior nasal nerve cryoablation, and septoplasty
- An understanding of essential office resources and pharmacology is needed for optimal results and to minimize risk of complications.

## INTRODUCTION

Over the past several years, the treatment of common rhinologic problems with in-office surgical procedures has increased dramatically in response to patient preferences, evolving insurance patterns, and changes in coding and reimbursement. Because this is an emerging practice, there has not been a lot of evidence published about how to best perform these techniques. This article provides practical advice from experienced surgeons related to the logistics and anesthetic techniques for conducting in-office surgical treatment of nasal airway obstruction. There may be alternative methods that may be equally or more effective, and the information provided herein is to help practitioners consider the issues involved in managing these patients perioperatively. These procedures can be performed reliably with excellent clinical outcomes as long as attention is paid to mitigate the potential clinical risks.

## BASIC OFFICE SET-UP

The procedures described can easily be performed in an office setting as long as specific logistical considerations are addressed. Minimum office resources include

Disclosure Statement: J. Atkins—Consultant for Arrinex and Acclarent. N. Bikhazi has nothing to disclose.

[a] Ogden Clinic, 4650 Harrison Boulevard, Ogden, UT 84403, USA; [b] Texas Sinus Center, 15900 La Cantera Parkway, Suite 20210, San Antonio, TX 78256, USA
* Corresponding author.
E-mail address: jatkins@texassinuscenter.com

1. An electric medical examination chair that allows a patient to recline in the event of a vagal episode
2. An endoscope tower, including monitor and light source and nasal/sinus operative instrumentation
   a. The specific instruments and their space requirements vary case by case.
   b. Ergonomics must be considered to allow a medical assistant or nurse to be in close proximity to the patient for monitoring and procedural assistance.

Additionally, the following equipment should be readily available in case of emergent problems:

1. A full cardiac monitor with ECG, blood pressure cuff, and pulse oximetry
2. An automated external defibrillator
3. Complete resuscitative equipment and medications, including
   A. Oxygen administered through a nasal cannula with a bag-valve mask bag present if a patient loses respiratory drive
   B. Intravenous (IV) set-up with accompanying fluids
   C. Epinephrine 1:1000 in case of anaphylaxis
   D. Naloxone for reversal of narcotics (can be given intramuscularly [IM] with autoinjector)[1]
   E. Flumazenil for reversal of benzodiazepines (requires placement of an IV for administration)[2]

Many of these procedures can be performed solely with topical and local anesthesia. Oral sedation may also be helpful particularly in cases of septoplasty or when these procedures are combined with more extensive procedures, such as office sinus surgery and/or balloon sinus dilation. If IV administered medication is needed, continual cardiopulmonary monitoring with a nurse/nurse anesthetist is required. Local/regional anesthesia techniques have several advantages over general anesthesia: preserving consciousness; reducing cardiovascular fluctuations, such as vasodilation and subsequent bleeding; and reducing respiratory depression and the stress response of surgery. This article primarily discusses the use of conscious sedation using local/topical anesthetics combined with oral sedatives and narcotics due to the excellent clinical results derived from these combinations of medications.

## LEGAL ISSUES AND LICENSURE

State licensing requirements for in-office procedural standards for anesthesia vary by state. Additionally, state requirements differ regarding orally administered narcotics and orally administered sedatives (conscious sedation) versus IV administered medication. Some states require that a physician register as providing office-based surgery whereas others do not. Moreover, notification of a malpractice carrier that in-office surgery is being performed is prudent to avoid potential issues.

The most common problems that occur during in-office procedures stem from the absence of the support infrastructure found in traditional surgical centers.[3] This is important because there are many potential safety hazards that office-based physicians are not used to considering—a review of patient medications; removal of personal items, such as cell phones or dentures; and review and monitoring of patient vital signs. One way to mitigate this risk is to treat office-based procedures similar to those performed in a surgical center. For example, a preoperative questionnaire similar to what is used in an ambulatory surgical center should be considered.

## PREPROCEDURE CLINICAL EVALUATION

In-office rhinologic procedures are not ideally suited for all patients. It is important to identify patients who will benefit from, and tolerate, the procedure. Excellent patients include those comfortable with oral sedation, with controllable anxiety, and with no significant fear of needles or injections. Surgeons should not rely on medications to allay patient fears or anxiety. For example, sedative/anxiolytics may, at times, have a paradoxic effect, disinhibiting a patient from controlling anxiety, leading to emotional lability and fear during the procedure. If these issues can be elucidated during patient selection, a clinician has a much more predictable outcome of success and the patient is more likely to be satisfied with the procedure.

Careful attention must be given to relevant medical comorbidities, which may raise the risk of office-based procedures. The American Society of Anesthesiologists (ASA) has identified medical classes that stratify surgical risk for patients on a scale of I to V. Although the exact ASA class is not necessarily a consideration for office-based procedures, an overall assessment of medical risk should be performed. Those patients with severe systemic illness, such as uncontrolled diabetes mellitus, coronary artery disease, uncontrolled hypertension, and severe pulmonary disease, should be moved to a more monitored setting with an anesthesiologist present. If a patient is on anticoagulation that needs to be stopped, this should be cleared with the primary physician/cardiologist prior to the procedure. Additionally, those patients receiving multiple medications should be monitored more closely due to potential drug interactions. Monitoring should be performed not only through the procedure but also for a period of time after the procedure to verify that the patient has had no subsequent respiratory or cardiovascular sequelae. Because the maximal effect of these medications is gradual and additive, this needs to be closely considered even after the procedure is completed.

The extent of anesthesia required should be tailored to patients, based on their comfort and the procedures that are going to be performed. More limited procedures may be accomplished solely with topical and or injected local anesthetics. More extensive procedures for nasal obstruction (such as septoplasty) or in patients who require multiple procedures, oral sedation, and/or analgesia may be make the procedure more tolerable.

## PHARMACOLOGIC AGENTS

Conscious sedation is the use of a combination of medications to help patients relax (a sedative) and to block pain (an anesthetic) during a medical or dental procedure (**Table 1**). Clinicians should consider topical applications of anesthetics and decongestants tantamount to systemic application due to the rapid absorptive capacity of the nasal mucosa. Specific contraindications to conscious sedation include pregnancy, severe alcoholism, glaucoma, or seizure disorder. These are based on the nonpredictable effects that medications used during conscious sedation may have on these associated comorbidities.

The goals of premedication are to reduce anxiety, provide mild sedation, provide analgesia, produce amnesia, and reduce anesthetic requirements. Allowance must be given for the time required for onset of medications; between 30 minutes and 60 minutes is needed for absorption after initial oral administration.

### Oral Anxiolytics/Sedatives

Benzodiazepines are widely used medications for the management of perioperative procedures via conscious sedation. Their chief advantage of oral administration is a

**Table 1**
**Common systemic and topical medications for office-based procedures**

| Medication Name | Dose | Onset/Duration of Action | Considerations |
|---|---|---|---|
| **Anxiolytics** | | | |
| Diazepam | 5–20 mg | Onset: 30–60 min | • Paradoxic agitation, anger, fear, anxiety |
| Lorazepam | 1–3 mg | Onset: 60–90 min | • Use with caution in patients with sleep apnea |
| | | | • Potential drug interactions, especially if patient using other sedating medications |
| | | | • Flumazenil for overdose |
| **Oral pain medication** | | | |
| Hydrocodone-acetaminophen | 5–20 mg of narcotic component based on patient's weight | Onset: 60 min | • Side effects: nausea, headache, drowsiness |
| Oxycodone-acetaminophen | | | • Allergic reactions ranging from urticarial to anaphylaxis |
| | | | • Interactions with other medications |
| | | | • Naloxone for overdose |
| **Topical decongestants** | | | |
| Phenylephrine | Soaked pledget | Onset: 2–3 min with maximum decongestion after 20 min Duration: 30 min–2.5–4 h | • α-Agonist • Shorter duration of action |
| Oxymetazoline | Soaked pledget | Onset: 2–3 min with maximum decongestion after 5–10 min Duration: 5–6 h | • α-Agonist • Longer duration of action • Best safety profile |
| Epinephrine | Soaked pledget | | • α-Agonist and β-agonist • Very potent vasoconstrictor • Can be irritating to the mucosa at high concentrations • Headache and hypertension in patients on β-blockers due to unopposed α stimulation |
| **Anesthetics** | Maximum dose | Duration | |
| Lidocaine | 4.5 mg/kg (7 with epinephrine) | 0.75–1.5 h | • Readily available • Can be obtained in a gel for precise topical application • Amide anesthetic |
| Cocaine | 3 mg/kg | 0.5–1 h | • Commercially available • Expensive • Requires stringent documentation/storage • Decongestant and anesthetic properties • Should not be injected • Ester anesthetic |

(*continued on next page*)

| Table 1 (continued) | | | |
|---|---|---|---|
| Medication Name | Dose | Onset/Duration of Action | Considerations |
| Tetracaine | 3 mg/kg | 1.5–6 h | • Less expensive<br>• Can be compounded into a gel<br>• Less documentation<br>• Should not be injected<br>• Ester anesthetic |

controlled and gradual anxiolytic and sedative-hypnotic effect. IV administration, which is not routinely used in office-based rhinologic procedures, requires the use of continual blood pressure and respiratory monitoring and is not discussed. These drugs also have the advantage of inducing periprocedure amnesia. The 2 main drugs used in this setting are diazepam (Valium) and lorazepam (Ativan). Typical preprocedure dosages are diazepam, 5 mg to 20 mg, or lorazepam, 1 mg to 3 mg. Diazepam has a fast onset after oral administration (within 30–60 minutes) whereas lorazepam takes slightly longer. These timing factors should be considered in preprocedure administration.

Paradoxic reactions, such as agitation, anger, fear, and anxiety, have been described and need to be considered if relaxation is not achieved. Care must also be taken in patients with sleep apnea to avoid worsening airway obstruction after the procedure is done. Although this class of medications rarely interacts with other medications, any drug that induces sedation or cognitive depression can be worsened by coadministration of benzodiazepines. Specifically, antihistamines found in many cough medications and other over-the-counter products can interact with these medications. Additionally, benzodiazepines are eliminated by the liver, so severe liver dysfunction can affect their pharmacologic elimination resulting in higher circulating levels and potential toxicity. Diazepam has the longest elimination among this group of agents (half-life of more than 100 hours) whereas lorazepam has an intermediate half-life of 10 hours to 20 hours. The potential for drug interactions must be considered in patients who use antidepressants, alcohol, and sleep medication after the procedure. Most commonly, respiratory support is needed in cases of oversedation and may include jaw thrust, oxygen administration, and, more severely, assisted ventilation. Flumazenil, a reversal agent, is now available for benzodiazepine oversedation but requires IV administration.

## Opioids

The goal of using narcotic agents is to initiate preemptive analgesia through a multi-modal approach.[4] Multimodality involves working on several different pathways to reduce perceived pain. Through preprocedure dosing, opioid receptors can be bound prior to nociceptive stimulus, resulting in diminished pain perception. Most commonly, hydrocodone or oxycodone in combination with acetaminophen is used at doses ranging from 5 mg to 20 mg based on patient weight. A graduated opioid dosing can be performed, but enough time should be allowed for oral absorption (at least 60 minutes) prior to the procedure. The most common side effects include nausea, headache, and drowsiness. Allergic reactions to opioids are common and can range most mildly from urticaria to, more severely, anaphylaxis.

Particular attention is needed when opioids are combined with other anxiolytic/sedatives. Opioid absorption is slow and toxicity is infrequent, but drug interactions and their additive sedation effects necessitate close monitoring. In particular, patients taking antihistamines, antidepressants, anxiolytics, and anticonvulsants need lower dosing and closer monitoring of opioids. This class of medication is also cleared through the liver and severe liver disease may reduce elimination and enhance toxicity. Naloxone, which can be administered through an IM autoinjectable dosing, is now readily available and should be kept on hand to reverse a patient who is suspected to have signs of oversedation. In case naloxone is administered, pulse oximetry and cardiac monitoring should be performed and hospital transfer considered.

### Compounded Agents

Compounded agents, such as 2% tetracaine solution combined with a topical decongestant and 4% tetracaine gel, are commonly used in office-based rhinology and offer several distinct advantages to the clinician. These agents can be tailored in potency to elicit excellent effects of anesthesia and decongestion. They are often combined into 1 solution, which is more time-efficient for application. Additionally, most clinicians are familiar with them because they are often used in the clinic setting and their physiologic effect is well-known. Some of the medications discussed later are compounded agents.

The reason these medications need to be obtained from a compounding pharmacy is because they are not mass produced or commercially available in a prepackaged format. Because these agents are customized and prepared in a compounding pharmacy, they are not considered Food and Drug Administration approved. Their safety, effectiveness, and manufacturing quality are not verified by the Food and Drug Administration. Oversight for compounding pharmacies rests with state pharmacy boards. Although most compounding pharmacies do an excellent job, it is incumbent on clinicians to be aware of the source of the compounded medications and to be aware of potential variations in potency and other quality-related issues.

### Topical Decongestants

Topical decongestants are sympathomimetics. Their action is mediated by stimulation of $\alpha$-receptors on smooth muscles, resulting in vasoconstriction of blood vessels. The 2 most common topical decongestants include oxymetazoline and phenylephrine. As discussed previously, these are often compounded with topical anesthetics in the form of a nasal spray that can be sprayed directly onto the nasal membranes or placed on cotton pledgets into the nose. Adequate time needs to be given for these agents to work, often up to 20 minutes. Both these agents are easy to use and have minimal toxicity but may include mild elevations in blood pressure and heart rate.

Although topical epinephrine is a potent vasoconstrictor, caution needs to be exercised when used in any concentration in the office. New adopters of in-office procedures need to use extreme caution when using epinephrine as a vasoconstrictor because of the potential disastrous effects of inadvertent injection of a 1:1000 concentration. As a firm rule, only a surgeon is allowed to draw up this medication and the needle is discarded immediately to avoid confusion. It can then be placed sparingly on a cottonoid (damp, not saturated). Epinephrine is effective at controlling epistaxis from sinus or septal tissue.

Even when topical epinephrine is appropriately diluted, if it is applied to an area not sufficiently vasoconstricted with oxymetazoline, a severe headache can occur associated with an increase in blood pressure. As discussed previously, any patient on $\beta$-blockers may have unmitigated $\alpha$ response to the epinephrine, and diastolic blood pressures can range as high as 140 mm Hg.

## Anesthetics

Anesthetic agents are the mainstay of operative anesthesia through their sensory blocking effects on peripheral nerves. The intention is to widely anesthetize the nasal membranes and bony structures to facilitate patient comfort during the procedure. Two broad classes are differentiated on their chemical side linkage: the amides (lidocaine, bupivacaine, prilocaine, procaine, and so forth) and the esters (benzocaine, cocaine, tetracaine, and so forth). Overall, the amide anesthetics like lidocaine—easily remembered by the fact that the names of medications in this family contain 2 "i"s—are much more commonly used in clinical practice due to their more favorable side-effect profile. Patients reporting allergy during dental procedures with procaine (Novocain) injection can be reassured that they are not at risk for allergic reaction with lidocaine because it belongs to a different drug class. True allergic reactions to Novocain/procaine were common in dental procedures because ester anesthetics are metabolized into para-aminobenzoic acid, which can elicit an allergic reaction. This is not the case with the amide anesthetics. True allergy to amide anesthetics is rare.[5] Some patients, however, may experience allergy to preservatives in amide anesthetic preparations. If there is clinical suspicion, skin testing can be done to confirm presence or absence of sensitivity.

## Topical Anesthetics

Topical anesthesia is paramount to success of office-based rhinology procedures. Total anesthetic agents can be combined with topical decongestants and left in place on the nasal mucosa to create excellent preprocedure anesthesia. The key to effective topical and local anesthesia is allowing the medications enough time to work prior to intervention. Although there are many topical anesthetics; those commonly used for in-office nasal procedures include 2% tetracaine or 4% cocaine.[6] Maximal dosing of both agents is 3 mg/kg and both these anesthetics should never be injected (which can result in significant cardiovascular compromise) but rather only be placed topically on the nasal mucosa. These medications should be use carefully in patients with uncontrolled hypertension, cardiac disease, known allergy to anesthetics, or neurologic impairment. Signs of toxicity of both agents may include lightheadedness, shallow breathing, tremors, headache, dizziness, and confusion.

Relative advantages/disadvantages of these medications include the following. The advantages of tetracaine:

1. Less regulation compared with cocaine
2. Can be used as a liquid or compounded into a gel
3. Less expensive than cocaine

The disadvantages of tetracaine:

1. Use of tetracaine alone without local anesthetic may result in a large amount of mucus drainage during the procedure. This seems to be attributed to patient underlying disease.
2. When compounded into a gel, inconsistent viscosity of the gel is common.
3. It usually needs to be combined with a topical vasoconstrictor, such as oxymetazoline or phenylephrine, which can lead to mixing errors.

The advantages of 4% cocaine:

1. Because it is manufactured, no mixing is needed, yielding consistent concentrations.
2. There is no noticed increase in mucus production when using topical cocaine.

The disadvantages of 4% cocaine:

1. It is more expensive than tetracaine.
2 It requires a double lock system.
3. It has more stringent accountability standards, requiring documentation in a nar-cotics/sedative logbook.
4. A patient may test positive on a urinalysis. Clearance time in urine is variable but is usually 3 days to 4 days. Most employers conducting urinalysis include a medical use clause.
   a. Department of Defense urinalysis protocol involves a medical review for this reason.[7]

With local or topical anesthetic, there should be access within the facility to lipid infusion capabilities to treat toxicity. In addition to traditional resuscitative methods, the American Society of Regional Anesthesia and Pain Medicine recommends lipid infusion begin at the first signs of local anesthesia toxicity.[8,9] There are cases reports of lipid infusions being effective at controlling cocaine toxicity as well.[10]

### Local Anesthestics (Injectable)

Most commonly lidocaine (Xylocaine), an amide, is often used with the addition of epinephrine in a concentration of either 1:100,000 or 1:200,000 to reduce bleeding. Care should be taken on the resulting effects of epinephrine because it may cause tachycardia and hypertension. More specifically, in patients on β-blockers, epineph-rine in small doses is considered safe, but severe uncontrolled hypertension can occur with larger doses. If lidocaine is used plain (without epinephrine), the maximal dose is 3 mg/kg. The addition of epinephrine slows absorption and raises the maximal dose to 7 mg/kg. Duration of effect ranges from 30 minutes to 1 hour.

Certain medical comorbidities may affect the safety of administered lidocaine. Because lidocaine is cleared by the liver, liver disease may increase accumulation of lidocaine in the body enhancing toxicity. Also, because lidocaine is protein bound, severe renal disease may reduce circulating protein increasing available drug, result-ing in toxicity. Additionally, patients on β-blockers or antibiotics may experience drug interactions with lidocaine, increasing the likelihood of toxicity. Toxicity may include clinical signs of lightheadedness, dizziness, tinnitus, visual disturbance, and head-ache. More severe signs include seizure, hypotension, bradycardia or tachycardia, and respiratory depression. In advanced reactions, immediate ventilation with 100% oxygen, cardiovascular resuscitation, and immediate ambulance transfer to a hospital is required.

Another injectable anesthetic bupivacaine (Marcaine) has a much longer duration of effect of up to 5 hours but is cardiotoxic and should be avoided as an injectable during office-based procedures.

## PREOPERATIVE TECHNIQUE FOR OFFICE-BASED PROCEDURES

Patients who require oral sedation are instructed to take the oral narcotic and oral anxiolytic medications 1 hour prior to the procedure. Commonly, hydrocodone or oxy-codone/acetaminophen is used as an oral narcotic, and lorazepam or diazepam is used as a sedative/anxiolytic agent. Dosage varies based on weight, medical condi-tion, age, and overall anxiety of the patient. Dosages range from 5 mg to 20 mg of hydrocodone/acetaminophen and 1 mg to 3 mg of lorazepam; 30 minutes prior to arrival, the patient self-administers oxymetazoline at the office, 2 squirts on each side, 3 separate times, with each application spaced 5 minutes to 10 minutes apart.

On arrival, front desk personnel should verify that the patient has a driver and ensures that the driver stays in the waiting room during the procedure. They also verify surgical consent and confirm the use of oxymetazoline, and, if the patient has not used oxymetazoline, it is administered during in-office preoperatively.

The medical assistant/nurse conducts a review of initial vital signs, provides the patient with postprocedure instructions, reviews them with the patient and the driver, and finally sprays the patient's nose with a topical anesthetic/decongestant (4% topical lidocaine/oxymetazoline or 2% tetracaine/phenylephrine solution).

The physician then assesses the patient and performs a time-out with the patient and the preoperative staff. The physician then administers 0.5 mL of oxymetazoline on each side directly onto the area being treated under endoscopic guidance using an LMA MADgic Laryngo-Tracheal Mucosal Atomization Device (Teleflex, Westmeath, Ireland).[11] Alternatively, medication can be applied to the desired area using pledgets. This ensures that the area to be treated is sufficiently vasoconstricted.

### Intraoperative Technique

Variation exists among clinicians performing office-based procedures regarding the routine use of cardiopulmonary monitoring. When a patient is significantly sedated, continuous monitoring should be used. Monitoring may include pulse oximetry, blood pressure, and ECG monitoring. The preferred means of local anesthesia is administration of 1% lidocaine with concentrations of epinephrine ranging from 1:100,000 to 1:200,000. The lower dose of epinephrine results in adequate vasoconstriction with less associated tachycardia. Although tachycardia from intranasal injections is transient, minimizing tachycardia is particularly important for awake patients because they may misperceive this effect as enhanced anxiety or as a complication of the procedure. One issue with local anesthesia is injecting it into the nasal tissue while avoiding inadvertent spillage down a patient's throat. For this reason, topical anesthetic alone can be used in selected patients. Recently, Entellus Medical (Stryker, Kalamazoo, MI) has released a needle to facilitate the injection of local anesthetic minimizing unintended extravasation down the throat. The needle is a 27-gauge needle with a reinforcing sleeve that supports the needle to reduce flexing during injection. The 27-gauge tip extends 2 mm in length with the reinforced portion acting as a backstop. Limiting the needle to 2 mm of penetration allows for even distribution of anesthetic without excess spillage (**Fig. 1**).

### Postoperative Technique

Final vital signs are taken and the patient is observed for up to 30 minutes for any sign of bleeding or medication side effect. If patients have taken a narcotic or sedative, they are taken by wheelchair to the car, and staff confirms they are leaving with a driver.

Topical anesthetics and 1:1000 epinephrine can irritate the mucosa once the anesthetic wears off. Some patients find the irritation more painful than the postoperative

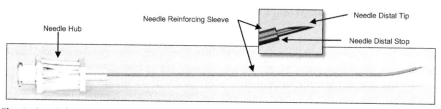

**Fig. 1.** Specialized needle for intranasal injections. Instructions for use: Entellus Medical Reinforced Anesthesia Needle US-3610-001 rA. (*Courtesy of* Entellus Medical, Inc, Plymouth, MN; with permission.)

pain of the procedure. Instructing patients to rinse their nose with a saline flush when they arrive home and again 30 minutes later eliminates this irritation. Patients are instructed to blow their nose after flushing, without obstructing one side or the other. Patients then continue routine saline rinses over the next week until they return.

## SPECIFIC OFFICE-BASED PROCEDURES
### Inferior Turbinate Surgery

There are 2 basic ways to reduce the size of the inferior turbinates—submucosal ablation and submucosal bone resection. Both of these can be performed safely with excellent patient satisfaction in the office and rarely require oral sedation when performed alone.

Submucosal ablation is less invasive than submucosal resection and can be accomplished routinely without injections. Ten minutes after application of topical lidocaine/oxymetazoline spray preoperatively, 2 full-size ½-inch × 3-inch cottonoids saturated with compounded 4% tetracaine gel are placed into each nostril, layering 1 cottonoid on top of the other, and verifying that they cover the inferior turbinate. These are left in place for 10 minutes. Laser or radiofrequency ablation devices can then be used to reduce the submucosal tissue. Outfracture of the inferior turbinates after the ablation can easily be performed using a Cottle elevator or Boies elevator. Most patients tolerate the outfracture well. Patients mention, however, that the sound of the outfracture can be startling. There can be a small amount of bleeding from the insertion site the application of cotton saturated with oxymetazoline or phenylephrine for an additional 10 minutes.

A similar protocol is used for submucosal bone resection conducted by a microdébrider shaver blade. After removal of the cottonoids, each inferior turbinate is injected with 1% lidocaine/1:200,000 epinephrine. The patients tolerate the microdébrider resection procedure well. The sound of the shaver can be alarming so it is important to warn them ahead of time. As with submucosal ablation, bilateral inferior turbinate outfracture after submucosal resection can be performed. Again, bleeding is controlled anteriorly with a cotton pledget soaked in topical decongestant.

### Nasal Valve Repair with Latera

Patients undergoing nasal valve repair with Latera in-office may receive an oral narcotic and oral sedative, but there is no need for intranasal decongestion or topical anesthesia preoperatively. This procedure can be relatively painless, but there are a couple of key points to minimize pain.

Applying a topical anesthetic benzocaine gel or tetracaine gel to the nasal vestibule for 10 minutes to 15 minutes prior to injection can help reduce the discomfort of the alar rim injections.

A sublabial block of the infraorbital nerve on each side can also be performed to enhance the anesthesia. To perform the block, a dental roll covered with 4% tetracaine gel is placed over the sublabial injection site for about 5 minutes to 10 minutes before starting the injection. A 25-gauge needle is used with 1% lidocaine/1:200,000 epinephrine infiltrating to the medial side of the infraorbital nerve creating a field block for the nose. This also takes 10 minutes to 15 minutes to take affect.

Once the alar rim is sufficiently numb, a 27-gauge or 30-gauge needle is used to anesthetize the alar rim insertion site and deployment tract. A minimum amount of lidocaine/1:200,000 epinephrine (0.25–0.5 mL) should be used in the tract as its purpose is to provide vasoconstriction/anesthesia. Hydrodissection of the tract should be avoided.

The cannula and subsequent deployment of the Latera stent is well-tolerated among these patients.

### Posterior Nasal Nerve Cryoablation with ClariFix

ClariFix (Arrinex, Redwood City, California) is a new device to perform posterior nasal nerve cryoablation in patients with chronic rhinitis. Lidocaine with oxymetazoline spray is applied preoperatively and allowed to sit for 10 minutes; ½-in × 3-in cottonoids are then trimmed to approximately 1-in length and saturated with a mixture of tetracaine/epinephrine, tetracaine/oxymetazoline, or 4% cocaine and placed in the inferior and middle meatuses. Pledgets should be placed posteriorly enough to abut the horizontal portion of the middle turbinate. Two pledgets are placed in each middle meatus with an additional full length ½-in × 3-in cottonoid saturated with tetracaine gel or cocaine placed on the superior surface of the inferior turbinate. Although the actual site of the cryoablation is farther posterior, part of the tubing supplying the nitrous oxide to the delivery tip of the device can become very cool. This tubing sometimes overlies the superior portion of the inferior turbinate, making it important to make sure this area is anesthetized.

Some surgeons apply lidocaine/oxymetazoline spray and then inject the area to be treated with 1% lidocaine/1:200,000 epinephrine instead of placing cottonoids into the nose. Both techniques seem to work equally well.

### Septoplasty

From a patient tolerance, septoplasty can be performed under local anesthesia in selected patients. Patients with more extensive bony/cartilaginous deviations may be more appropriate for general anesthesia. Limited anterior deviation or localized bony/cartilaginous spurs are ideal for the in-office approach.

The septum is topically anesthetized with preoperative anesthetic/decongestant solution. After 10 minutes, cottonoids with tetracaine or cocaine are placed onto the septum before injecting 1% lidocaine/1:100,000 epinephrine. Standard injections are performed in a similar manner as those performed in the operating room. Depending on the anatomic variation of the septum, some patients need a standard submucosal resection. Patients who have an isolated but significant bone spur occasionally requires only the use of a septal burr from one of the major shaver manufacturers. Use of the septal burr in an awake patient is more troubling to patients than a submucosal resection. Their discomfort is not from pain, but because vibrations from the shaver tend to radiate into their temporal bone, which patients describe as annoying. For this reason, the authors typically perform a standard submucosal resection.

Conducting septoplasty in-office requires more training for the individuals assisting the surgeon. Conversely, most other procedures, discussed previously, and most balloon sinus dilation procedures performed in-office require only a surgeon with little help from an assistant. Septoplasty with submucosal resection requires trained individual to assist, which may complicate offering this procedure on a routine basis. Hiring a surgical technician to work in-office on days that have a septoplasty scheduled can be helpful. Performing a submucosal resection endoscopically yields no incremental costs to the procedure because endoscopes are available in the office; however, a traditional nonendoscopic submucosal resection requires a good headlight, adding some upfront costs to septoplasty.

## FINANCIAL CONSIDERATIONS

Primarily, performance of office-based rhinologic procedures affords an improved financial reward to patients, with reduced copay, lack of anesthesia and facility fees, and a faster time to return to work.[12] Additionally, there may be scheduling efficiencies for the surgeon performing these procedures in the office rather than in an operating room or ambulatory surgery center setting.

There are important financial aspects to consider for each one of these procedures performed independently. When multiple procedures are performed, the reimbursement for some procedures is considerably less due to multiprocedure reimbursement policies.

Submucosal ablation of the inferior turbinates with either a laser or radiofrequency involves the up-front cost of the device and a per-case cost for the disposable handpiece. The reimbursement for this procedure tends to be low and it takes many cases to recover the capital cost of the main device. Adding this procedure to other rhinologic procedures, however, such as balloon sinus dilation, can help cover of the cost of submucosal ablation.

Submucosal resection of the inferior turbinate bone yields greater reimbursement than submucosal tissue ablation. Compared with reimbursement for submucosal resection of the inferior turbinates, the cost for a mechanical turbinate shaving device is significantly more expensive. The use of reusable shaver blades amortized over the number of uses is an option to make this procedure more financially feasible. Also, as of January 1, 2018, the global period for submucosal resection of the inferior turbinates has gone from 90 days to 0 days, allowing for some reimbursement in the postoperative period.

Latera and posterior nerve cryoablation require disposable devices and the reimbursement varies based on an individual provider's contract. With patient volume, purchasing in bulk may help reduce the supply costs of these procedures.

Reimbursement for septoplasty is low enough that it rarely justifies being conducted as a standalone in-office procedure. Nonetheless, in-office septoplasty can be helpful for accessing the sinuses for balloon sinus dilation or sinus surgery. There are no device costs, but the up-front costs of a septoplasty tray can be expensive. The per-case procedure costs of suture and septal splints add to the overhead of the case as well. The potential difficulty of the procedure may lead the clinician to defer some septoplasty to the operating room.

## SUMMARY

In summary, procedures for nasal airway obstruction can be safely and comfortably conducted in the office setting. The standard for clinical success of in-office procedures should be the same as those performed under general anesthesia with the additional advantages of quicker recovery and improved economics for the patient and health care system. An increase in patient satisfaction yields an all-around improved experience relative to the procedures being performed in the operating room. A detailed understanding of in-office procedural process, medications, and risks can facilitate adoption of these innovative strategies.

## REFERENCES

1. DailyMed - NALOXONE HYDROCHLORIDE- naloxone hydrochloride injection, solution. Available at: https://dailymed.nlm.nih.gov/dailymed/drugInfo.cfm?setid=307ae923-3c84-4844-9bbb-c5c5528623ac. Accessed January 13, 2018.
2. DailyMed - FLUMAZENIL- flumazenil injection. Available at: https://dailymed.nlm.nih.gov/dailymed/drugInfo.cfm?setid=cf39cdaf-8cb7-4dbb-8672-9cf8e91ac86c. Accessed January 13, 2018.
3. Shapiro FE, Punwani N, Rosenberg NM, et al. Office-based anesthesia: safety and outcomes. Anesth Analg 2014;119(2):276–85.

4. Vadivelu N, Mitra S, Schermer E, et al. Preventive analgesia for postoperative pain control: a broader concept. Local Reg Anesth 2014;7:17–22.

5. Koda-Kimble MA, Young LY. Applied therapeutics: the clinical use of drugs. 6th edition. Baltimore (MD): Lippincott Williams & Wilkins; 2001. p. 11–3. Chicago.

6. DailyMed - COCAINE HYDROCHLORIDE- cocaine hydrochloride solution. Available at: https://dailymed.nlm.nih.gov/dailymed/drugInfo.cfm?setid=24faa247-fe12-4574-881d-445b078b3e87. Accessed January 13, 2018.

7. DoD Instruction 1010.16: Technical Procedures for the Military Drug Abuse Testing Program, Defense Department Office of the Under Secretary for Personnel and Readiness. Available at: https://prhome.defense.gov/Portals/52/Documents/RFM/Readiness/DDRP/docs/1%20DODI%201010.16%20Drug%20Lab%20Technical%20Procedures.pdf. Accessed June 22, 2018.

8. Local Anesthetic Toxicity Treatment & Management: Approach Considerations, Treatment of Central Nervous System Toxicity, Treatment of Cardiovascular Toxicity. 2017. Available at: https://emedicine.medscape.com/article/1844551-treatment. Accessed January 13, 2018.

9. Asra_last_checklist_2018.pdf. Available at: https://www.asra.com/content/documents/asra_last_checklist_2018.pdf. Accessed January 13, 2018.

10. Jakkala-Saibaba R, Morgan PG, Morton GL. Treatment of cocaine overdose with lipid emulsion. Anaesthesia 2011;66(12):1168–70.

11. Teleflex, Anesthesia and Respiratory Catalog, LMA Madgic Laryngo-Tracheal Mucosal Atomization Device. Available at: https://www.teleflexarcatalog.com/anesthesia-respiratory/airway/category/lma-sup-reg-sup-madgic-sup-reg-sup-laryngo-tracheal-mucosal-atomization-device. Accessed June 17, 2018.

12. Bikhazi N, Light J, Truitt T, et al. REMODEL: standalone balloon dilation versus sinus surgery for chronic rhinosinusitis: a prospective, multicenter, randomized, controlled trial with 1-year follow-up. Am J Rhinol Allergy 2014;28(4):323–9.

# Pediatric Nasal Obstruction

Matthew M. Smith, MD[a], Stacey L. Ishman, MD, MPH[b,c],*

## KEYWORDS

- Nasal obstruction • Choanal atresia • Pyriform aperture stenosis • Rhinitis
- Rhinosinusitis • Juvenile angiofibroma

## KEY POINTS

- Newborns with bilateral congenital nasal obstruction will present very early to the physician with desaturations with feeding.
- Nasal dermoids, gliomas, and encephaloceles are the most common causes of midline nasal masses. A positive Furstenberg sign is diagnostic of an encephalocele.
- Chronic rhinosinusitis and allergic rhinitis overlap significantly and, untreated, can lead to a significant decrease in quality of life.
- Intervention is always needed for removal of nasal foreign bodies to prevent further migration into the esophagus or the larynx, precipitating an airway emergency.
- Anterior bowing of the posterior maxillary wall, along with widening of the sphenopalatine foramen, are hallmark radiologic signs of a juvenile angiofibroma.

## INTRODUCTION

Pediatric nasal obstruction is one of the most common problems seen by pediatric otolaryngologists. Typically, this is not an urgent diagnosis but is more commonly associated with reduced quality of life. However, prompt treatment of nasal obstruction can be critical in newborns and infants because of their obligatory nasal breathing. A variety of congenital causes for pediatric nasal obstruction, including choanal atresia, pyriform aperture stenosis, and midline nasal masses can present with respiratory or feeding complaints. As children get older, inflammatory and infectious causes of nasal obstruction are more common and lead to significantly reduced

Disclosure: Dr M.M. Smith has nothing to disclose. Dr S.L. Ishman is a consultant for Medtronic.
[a] Department of Pediatric Otolaryngology, Cincinnati Children's Hospital Medical Center, 3333 Burnet Avenue, MLC 2018, Cincinnati, OH 45229, USA; [b] Department of Otolaryngology, Upper Airway Center, Cincinnati Children's Hospital Medical Center, University of Cincinnati, 3333 Burnet Avenue, MLC 2018, Cincinnati, OH 45229, USA; [c] Department of Pulmonary Medicine, Upper Airway Center, Cincinnati Children's Hospital Medical Center, University of Cincinnati, 3333 Burnet Avenue, MLC 2018, Cincinnati, OH 45229, USA
* Corresponding author. Department of Otolaryngology, Upper Airway Center, Cincinnati Children's Hospital Medical Center, University of Cincinnati, 3333 Burnet Avenue, MLC 2018, Cincinnati, OH 45229.
E-mail address: Stacey.Ishman@cchmc.org

quality of life and increased health care expenditures. Within this article, the authors discuss the approach and workup of a child with nasal obstruction, along with a description of commonly encountered causes.

## HISTORY

As with other disease processes, obtaining an accurate history, including laterality, is very important to narrow the differential diagnoses (**Box 1**) for nasal obstruction. Newborns with bilateral congenital nasal obstruction will present soon after birth with desaturations or blue spells because they are unable to coordinate feeding and breathing. Left untreated, this results in failure to thrive. Unilateral congenital nasal obstruction typically presents later in life, as feeding is typically not significantly impeded. Birth history, including Apgar scores; family history (including any atopy); parental pregnancy history, including exposure to teratogens; response to allergens; and complete past medical and surgical histories will assist the clinician when narrowing down the differential.

## PHYSICAL EXAMINATION

The physical examination should begin with observation for retractions, nasal flaring, visible nasal obstructive masses or other midline defects, and the presence of mouth breathing. If there are signs of respiratory distress, such as cyanosis, labored breathing, or substernal or subcostal retractions, airway management should be initiated. This management may include supplemental oxygen, noninvasive ventilation, or even intubation. Management of feeding through a nasogastric tube may be required. In newborns, a 5F or 6F catheter is passed through the nasal cavity to establish the patency of the posterior choanae. It is important to see the catheter transorally in order to establish patency; the catheter can become coiled in the nasal cavity and seem to pass through the choanae without actually doing so. If there is concern for a skull base defect, and the catheter is not able to be passed, placing a mirror under the nares to check for condensation is a noninvasive evaluation of nasal patency. Anterior rhinoscopy is also useful to examine the septum, inferior and middle turbinates, internal nasal valve, and to assess for polyps or purulence. Flexible and/or rigid nasal endoscopy is very useful in determining the presence of nasal structural obstruction or masses. The ease and success of this evaluation is based on the cooperation of the child and permission of the parent.

## IMAGING

Computed tomography (CT) and/or MRI, alone or in combination, are the most common modalities used to assess pediatric nasal obstruction. CT is best used to evaluate the bony skeleton, and MRI is best used to evaluate the soft tissue as well as the extent of intracranial involvement. One advantage of MRI over CT is the lack of radiation exposure. However, in young or uncooperative children, sedation may be required. In pediatric patients who have undergone implant procedures (eg, cochlear implantation), CT is preferred to avoid displacing the implant.

## DIFFERENTIAL DIAGNOSIS

As demonstrated in **Box 1**, there are a multitude of causes for pediatric nasal obstruction. The authors discuss the most commonly encountered causes next.

**Box 1**
**Differential diagnosis of pediatric nasal obstruction**

Congenital
  Cleft lip nasal deformity
  Choanal atresia
  Dermoids
  Encephalocele
  Glioma
  Nasolacrimal duct cysts
  Pyriform aperture stenosis
  Thornwaldt cyst

Inflammatory/infectious
  Adenoid hypertrophy
  Allergic rhinitis
  Nonallergic rhinitis: with and without eosinophilia
  Rhinosinusitis: acute and chronic
  Inferior turbinate hypertrophy
  Nasal polyposis
  Vasomotor rhinitis
  Rhinitis medicamentosa

Neoplasms
  Benign
    Juvenile nasopharyngeal angiofibroma (JNA)
    Hemangioma
    Nasal dermoid
    Nasal osteoma
    Nasopharyngeal teratoma
    Neurofibroma
    Papilloma
    Salivary gland tumor: benign
  Malignant
    Adenocarcinoma
    Esthesioneuroblastoma
    Lymphoma
    Metastatic disease
    Nasopharyngeal carcinoma
    Rhabdomyosarcoma
    Squamous cell carcinoma
    Salivary gland tumor: malignant

Systemic
  Cystic fibrosis
  Primary ciliary dyskinesia
  Wegener granulomatosis
  Sarcoidosis

Trauma/iatrogenic
  Empty nose syndrome
  Nasal foreign body
  Nasal valve collapse: internal and external
  Postrhinoplasty nasal defects
  Septal deviation
  Silent sinus syndrome
  Synechiae

## CONGENITAL
### Choanal Atresia

Embryologically, there are 5 recognizable facial structures (frontonasal prominence, right and left maxillary prominence, and right and left mandibular prominence) that become evident around 4 weeks' gestational age.[1] Over the next few weeks, these prominences rotate to fuse in the midline. The nasal pits continue to invaginate toward the pharynx and oral cavity to create a connection between the nasal cavity and the pharynx during weeks 6 to 7. If the nasal cavity is not in continuity with the nasopharynx and/or oropharynx, then nasal breathing is significantly impaired. The nasobuccal membrane is a posterior barrier between the nasal cavity and pharynx. This membrane eventually obliterates; if it does not occur, choanal atresia is thought to result. A second theory regarding the development of choanal atresia suggests that it results from the persistence of the buccopharyngeal membrane, which normally obliterates to form a direct pathway between the oral cavity and the pharynx.[2]

The incidence of choanal atresia is low (1 in 5000–7000 live births), and most are unilateral.[3] With an almost 2:1 ratio, girls are more likely to have choanal atresia.[4] Choanal atresia can be classified into 3 types, bony, membranous, or bony-membranous, with the last type accounting for most cases.[5] Choanal atresia has been seen in association with many other craniofacial abnormalities, but the most common relationship is with CHARGE syndrome (coloboma, heart defects, choanal atresia, growth retardation, genitourinary abnormalities, ear abnormalities). CT is the preferred imaging modality to assess this disorder (**Fig. 1**).

Management differs for children with unilateral versus bilateral atresia. Bilateral atresia is a relative emergency because newborns are obligate nasal breathers. Nonsurgical strategies include the use of a McGovern nipple, oral airway placement

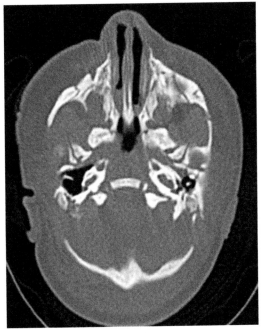

**Fig. 1.** CT demonstrating bilateral choanal atresia.

to displace the soft palate posteriorly, or endotracheal intubation.[6] Surgical management should be used as soon as feasible based on the medical status of the newborn. However, unilateral choanal atresia does not require urgent treatment, as these children do not present with feeding difficulties. In fact, it is common for these children to be misdiagnosed or undiagnosed until later in life. When properly identified, unilateral atresia is ideally fixed before 5 years of age in order to avoid persistent unilateral nasal drainage, which can be socially and medically problematic.

Surgical approaches to choanal atresia include the transnasal or transpalatal techniques. The sublabial technique is not discussed. The transnasal approach was popularized with the introduction of endoscopic nasal surgery. If the bony atretic plate is less than 3 mm in thickness, a transnasal approach is the most commonly recommended. A 0° endoscope is used transnasally with a simultaneous view of the nasopharynx through a transoral 120° endoscope. Urethral sounds can be used to puncture the atretic plate or, if the bony plate is thick, a drill can be used to puncture through the plate. It is important to use both the transnasal and transoral views in order to avoid potentially entering the anterior skull base. Following puncture of the atretic place, a drill is used to widen the choanae to the appropriate size. Because of the risk of restenosis and crusting at the site of the bony atresia, some physicians will advocate the use of a nasoseptal flap based off the posterior septal artery to lay over the bony edges following the removal of the atretic plate. Based on the preference of the physician, stents may then be placed and kept in place for 3 weeks or less. Complications include epistaxis or restenosis. A recent meta-analysis found similar success rates for bilateral choanal atresia repair regardless of whether stents were used.[7] In the transpalatal approach, which is currently rarely used, a W-shaped palatal flap is made that is supplied by the bilateral greater palatine arteries. After raising the flap, the portion of the palatine bone anterior to the vomer and the atretic plates are removed with a combination of a drill and rongeur. The atretic plates are then identified and removed along with the posterior septum. Stents (often small endotracheal tubes) may then be placed and the flap closed. Complications include restenosis of the choanae, palatal fistulas, or flap necrosis.[8]

### Pyriform Aperture Stenosis

Pyriform aperture stenosis, also known as anterior nasal stenosis, was first reported by Brown and colleagues,[9] who hypothesized that it resulted from bony overgrowth of the nasal process of the maxilla. The pyriform aperture is defined as the anterior most nasal inlet that is pear shaped and bounded by the nasal bones, nasal process of the maxilla, and horizontal process.[10] This portion is the narrowest of the nasal cavity. Patients with this condition will present with similar symptoms to those of children with bilateral choanal atresia with feeding difficulties and cyclical cyanosis relieved by crying. A review of 34 infants found the most common presenting signs and symptoms with congenital nasal obstruction were stertor (44%), cyanosis (24%), stridor (24%), retractions (21%), rhinorrhea (21%), apnea (12%), and epistaxis (8%), with 21% of infants having pyriform aperture stenosis.[11] CT is the imaging modality of choice, with typical findings including narrowing and inward bowing of the anterior nasal process[10] (**Fig. 2**). There is an association between the presence of a central mega-maxillary incisor, holoprosencephaly, and pyriform aperture stenosis. Airway management is again the most important aspect of treatment. Medical interventions include the use of a McGovern nipple, oral airway, or endotracheal intubation. When the distance between the pyriform apertures is less than 5.7 mm, a pooled case series reported an 88% sensitivity and specificity that surgical intervention would be required.[12]

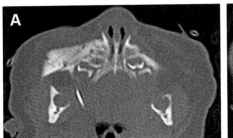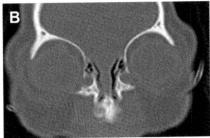

Fig. 2. (A) CT (axial) demonstrating bilateral pyriform aperture stenosis. (B) CT (coronal).

Surgical management of pyriform aperture stenosis typically involves a translabial incision made down through the mucosa and periosteum superior to the right canine tooth and extending to the left canine region. The soft tissue and periosteum are then elevated to expose the lateral nasal side wall, nasal floor, and the stenosis. Using a drill, the hypertrophic bone is then drilled down, taking care not to injure underlying tooth buds. The nasal mucosa is then draped back over the nasal floor, and nasal stents are placed. The sublabial incision is then closed and the stents kept in place for 2 to 6 weeks based on the physician's preference.

## Midline Nasal Masses

Understanding the fetal development of the midface and anterior skull base allows the physician to diagnose midline defects. Following the development of the neural tube and its closure, neural crest cells migrate into position adjacent to the mesenchyme. If fusion is incomplete, congenital midline nasal masses can result. The 3 most important spaces related to congenital midline nasal mass development are the fonticulus nasofrontalis, prenasal space, and the foramen cecum. The prenasal space is the area between the nasal bones and the nasal capsule and is the typical area for either external or internal manifestations of midline nasal lesions. The fonticulus nasofrontalis is the space between the frontal and nasal bones. If this space persists during development, it can serve as a direct pathway to the anterior skull base or a patent sinus tract. A patent fonticulus nasofrontalis will typically manifest as an external midline nasal lesion (**Fig. 3**). The foramen cecum is the area between the posterior boundary of the frontal bone and the anterior boundary of the ethmoid sinuses. It typically runs in the area that develops into the frontoethmoidal suture line. This line connects directly with the prenasal space and if left patent can allow direct access from the anterior skull base to the nasal cavity. A patent foramen cecum will typically manifest as an internal midline nasal lesion (see **Fig. 3**). Because of the potential intracranial attachments, all midline nasal masses can pose a threat of meningitis.

### Nasal dermoid cysts

Nasal dermoid cysts form from mesoderm and ectoderm components. They develop from ectodermal elements adhering to mesodermal elements (fibrous tissue) that are drawn posterosuperior through a patent prenasal space.[13] Dermoid cysts can lie anywhere along this persistent space, even attaching to dura in approximately 4% to 45% of cases.[14] Nasal dermoids can be visible externally as a midline nasal mass with a small tuft of hair or can distort the face without any evidence of a fistulous tract. Nasal dermoids do not enlarge and do not transilluminate. For midline nasal masses, MRI is typically the imaging modality of choice because of the decreased risk of radiation and improved imaging of the skull base.

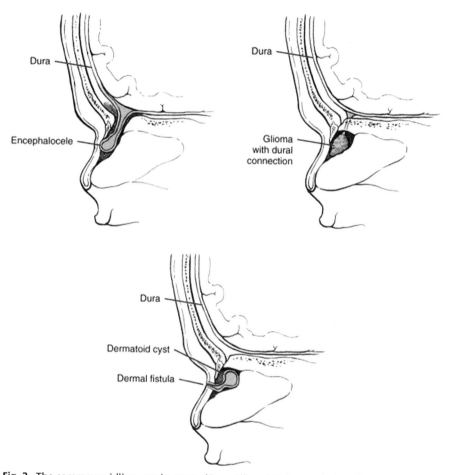

**Fig. 3.** The common midline nasal masses. (*From* Elluru RG. Congenital malformations of the nose and nasopharynx. In: Flint PW, Haughey BH, Lund V, et al, editors. Cummings otolaryngology. 6th edition. Philadelphia: Saunders; 2015. p. 2945; with permission.)

There are many different surgical approaches to remove nasal dermoids, but the 2 most common techniques are the external vertical midline incision and the open rhinoplasty approach. The vertical midline incision provides direct access to the dermoid but can leave a small but visible external scar over the nasal dorsum. The open rhinoplasty approach provides excellent exposure for access to the nasal bones in case the dermoid extends underneath the nasal bones. If there is a fistulous tract, then a combination of both approaches can be very useful to ensure complete removal of the dermoid. In addition, a small external incision can be made with endoscopic removal of the dermoid, especially if there is no intracranial extension.

### Gliomas

Gliomas result from extracranial glial tissue that travels outside the cranial vault via a patent fonticulus nasofrontalis. Gliomas can be extranasal, intranasal, or both with a rate of 6:3:1, respectively.[15] They typically present as a noncompressible, nontransilluminating nasal mass. They can present with a widened nasal dorsum, and the most common complaint is nasal obstruction. MRI is the imaging modality of choice.

Surgical treatment is typically through an intranasal, endoscopic approach. Identifying the base/stalk of the glioma and then amputating it is the primary surgical technique used. External approaches are rare but are dictated by the location of the mass itself. Having neurosurgical support on standby is advisable in the rare instance that there is noted to be intracranial extension that was not identified on preoperative imaging.

### Encephaloceles

Encephaloceles are composed of both glial and brain tissue and can also contain meninges (meningoencephalocele). These potential midline nasal masses occur from a persistent opening of the fonticulus nasofrontalis and/or the foramen cecum. Unlike nasal dermoids or gliomas, these masses enlarge with crying, straining, or external compression of the jugular vein (positive Furstenberg sign) and will transilluminate. MRI is the imaging modality of choice to identify the extent of brain tissue involved. Whenever brain contents are involved, the otolaryngologist should coordinate the surgical removal with a neurosurgeon. The location of the encephalocele will dictate the approach to the lesion, but many times a combined intranasal and intracranial approach is taken. Because of the connection to the cranial vault, the chance for postoperative cerebrospinal fluid leak is increased compared with gliomas and nasal dermoids.

### Tornwaldt cysts

Tornwaldt cysts are another midline nasopharyngeal mass that can cause nasal obstruction. First described as a pathologic entity by Tornwaldt in 1885, this uncommon mass develops as a nasopharyngeal cyst that usually sits just above the superior pharyngeal constrictor muscles, at the level of the fossa of Rosenmüller.[16] If there is evidence of nasal obstruction from a nasopharyngeal cyst, treatment typically consists of an intranasal, endoscopic approach to marsupialize the cyst.

### Nasolacrimal Duct Cysts

Nasolacrimal cysts develop from incomplete cannulation of the nasolacrimal duct during fetal development, which can cause significant nasal obstruction and respiratory distress in an infant.[17] These cysts present with significant epiphora secondary to obstruction of the lacrimal duct. Nasal endoscopy will demonstrate a cystic mass emanating from the inferior meatus, which may obscure the view of the inferior turbinate. CT is the imaging modality of choice. Depending on the severity of symptoms, treatment can vary from observation to surgical intervention. Ophthalmologists and otolaryngologists will generally work side by side during the surgery. The otolaryngologist will typically marsupialize the cyst endoscopically, followed by the cannulation of the lacrimal duct system by ophthalmology.

### Cleft Lip Nasal Deformity

Clefts of the lip and/or palate occur in around 1 per 800 births.[18] Physical deformities resulting from a cleft lip include a flattened nasal bridge, columellar displacement to the contralateral side, and a flattened nasal ala on the side of the cleft (**Fig. 4**). The flattened nasal ala is the result of an immature and weak alar cartilage that leads to collapse over the poorly formed premaxilla. In addition to the columellar displacement, the caudal septum can be deflected off of the maxillary crest, which can lead to a septal deviation. These nasal anatomic deformities can lead to significant nasal

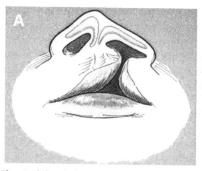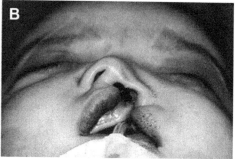

**Fig. 4.** (*A*) A left complete unilateral cleft and palate with obvious asymmetry of the alar base. (*B*) Base photograph of a left complete unilateral cleft and palate with obvious asymmetry of the alar base. (*From* Sykes JM, Jang YJ. Cleft lip rhinoplasty. Facial Plast Surg Clin North Am 2009;17(1):135; with permission.)

obstruction among those patients with a cleft lip. Farzal and colleagues[19] recently found that there was noted to be up to a 29% decrease in nasal volume among patients with a unilateral cleft lip. Surgical correction of the cleft lip followed by pediatric rhinoplasty (**Fig. 5**) can help to correct the nasal deformity, but it must be made clear to the patients that multiple surgeries may be needed to correct all the deformities.

## INFLAMMATORY/INFECTIOUS
### Allergic Rhinitis

Allergic rhinitis is one of the most common causes of pediatric nasal obstruction, which affects 8% to 16% of children and is immunoglobulin E mediated.[20,21]

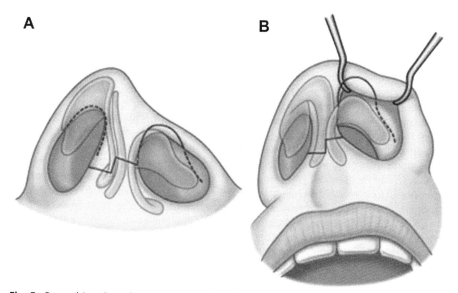

**Fig. 5.** Open rhinoplasty for secondary unilateral cleft nasal deformity. (*A*) Left cleft lip nasal deformity. (*B*) Proposed surgical realignment of nasal deformity. (*From* Chen PK, Noordhoff SM. Secondary cleft lip and cleft nasal deformity. In: Chung KC, Disa JJ, Gosain AK, et al, editors. Plastic surgery: indications and practice. Philadelphia: Saunders; 2009. p. 551; with permission.)

Children will typically complain of itchy and watery eyes, nasal obstruction, clear rhinorrhea, chronic fatigue, and sometimes cough. Depending on the duration of disease before treatment, children can become primary mouth breathers and develop facial abnormalities associated with mouth breathing and lack of nasal airflow.[22] Anterior rhinoscopy will usually reveal pale, boggy mucosa of the nasal cavity, inferior turbinate hypertrophy, and clear nasal secretions. No imaging is required in the workup of allergic rhinitis. Treatment is primarily medical and involves intranasal steroids, oral and intranasal antihistamines, leukotriene modifiers, and saline irrigation.[23] Targeted allergen therapy is also available if medical treatment is not adequate and typically involves immunotherapy. In addition to medical therapy, submucous resection of the inferior turbinates has been shown to be a safe and effective complementary treatment to relieve airway obstruction in these patients.[24]

### Chronic Rhinosinusitis

Chronic rhinosinusitis (CRS) is another clinical entity that results in a significant burden and decreased quality of life in children and overlaps with allergic rhinitis in up to 60% of patients.[25] Families of children with nasal obstruction secondary to rhinosinusitis have reported more limitations to daily activities than do parents of children with asthma.[26]

Clinical presentation includes persistent nasal drainage, nasal obstruction, and a change in smell/lack of smell for a duration of 3 months or greater. Nasal polyposis can also be present and cause significant nasal obstruction. In pediatric patients, the presence of nasal polyps should prompt the clinician to evaluate for cystic fibrosis. Although rare in children, antrochoanal polyps can also be present in the setting of CRS; removal of these can lead to significant improvement in nasal airflow. CT is the imaging modality of choice for CRS and can help identify other bony entities that might contribute to nasal obstruction, including concha bullosa, deviated septum, and inferior turbinate hypertrophy.

Traditional surgical treatments for CRS include adenoidectomy, maxillary sinus lavage, and functional endoscopic sinus surgery (FESS). Adenoidectomy is traditionally the first-line therapy for children who fail medication management of CRS. A 2008 meta-analysis of adenoidectomy for pediatric chronic sinusitis found that adenoidectomy alone improved patient or caregiver reports of symptom improvement in 69.3% overall (95% confidence interval = 56.8%–81.7%, $P<.001$).[27] Maxillary sinus lavage is less commonly used, although a 2008 study suggested that adenoidectomy with lavage was more effective than adenoidectomy alone for children with high Lund-Mackay sinus CT scores, whereas those with low scores did not benefit.[28] Another modality that has been gaining more popularity is balloon sinuplasty. A recent prospective, multicenter study demonstrated significant symptom improvement 6 months after dilation in children with CRS, without any reported complications.[29] If a child has extensive polyposis, then debridement of the polyps must be performed and balloon sinuplasty alone is inappropriate. FESS should be considered when medical therapy and adenoidectomy have failed or if there is a large burden of nasal polyps. Depending on the severity of disease, the comfort level of the physician, local resources, and previous surgical history, image guidance can be a valuable tool to provide the correct roadmap of the sino-nasal cavity in order to avoid damaging adjacent structures (orbit, anterior skull base, carotid artery, anterior ethmoid artery, optic nerve).

## TRAUMA/IATROGENIC
### Structural Nasal Defects

Whether from previous trauma or natural growth, another common cause of nasal obstruction is a deviated septum. Septal deviation rates, depending on the location of the deviation, range from 0.7% to 28.7% in children.[30] Nasal septal deviation is more prevalent in older children and adults, which may be due to the increased incidence of external trauma experienced later in life.[31] Regardless of the mechanism of injury, septoplasty has been advocated in children older than age 6; but recent reports have suggested that earlier septoplasty might help prevent dental malocclusion and other craniofacial abnormalities later in childhood.[32] Other types of nasal trauma can also present with nasal obstruction, such as nasal bone fracture, septal hematoma, or septal abscess. Septal hematomas and abscesses are typically drained, either under local anesthesia or in the operating room. Septoplasty is performed under general anesthesia with most experts advocating that bony septal work be delayed until after puberty.

### Nasal Foreign Bodies

More common in younger children, nasal foreign bodies must always be on the differential of nasal obstruction in children. Intervention is always needed for nasal foreign body removal in order to prevent further migration distally, potentially precipitating an airway emergency. The timing of removal is often based on the foreign body involved. Batteries are always considered an emergency because of the complications associated with prolonged exposure (septal perforation, saddle nose deformity, orbital injury, synechiae). However, nasal foreign bodies can often be removed without general anesthesia if the child is cooperative.

## NEOPLASMS
### Juvenile Nasopharyngeal Angiofibroma

Juvenile nasopharyngeal angiofibromas present with recurrent epistaxis and unilateral nasal obstruction. They are only seen in males and typically present during adolescence. Even though this is considered a benign tumor, it can be very locally destructive. Nasal endoscopy will reveal a vascular mass near the posterior attachment of the middle turbinate, at the opening of the sphenopalatine foramen. Imaging can reveal (**Fig. 6**) an anterior bowing of the posterior maxillary sinus wall (Holman-Miller sign). Before surgical intervention, embolization is typically performed to decrease the vascularity of the tumor. Blood should be typed and screened before arrival to the operating room because of the high likelihood of blood loss (often 500–1000 mL or higher). Both endoscopic and open approaches have been advocated, and the approach is generally dictated based on the location and size of the mass along with the preference and comfort of the surgeon.

### Nasopharyngeal Teratomas

Teratomas are benign neoplasms that are formed from an abnormal development of all 3 germ layers (ectoderm, mesoderm, endoderm) resulting in a soft tissue mass. When located within the nasopharynx, these masses can be potentially life threatening if there is both nasopharyngeal and oropharyngeal compromise leading to respiratory distress. It is imperative to have both a CT and MRI before proceeding with surgery to determine if there is any connection with the anterior skull base (**Fig. 7**). A combination of transoral and transnasal approaches are typically used to remove these masses.

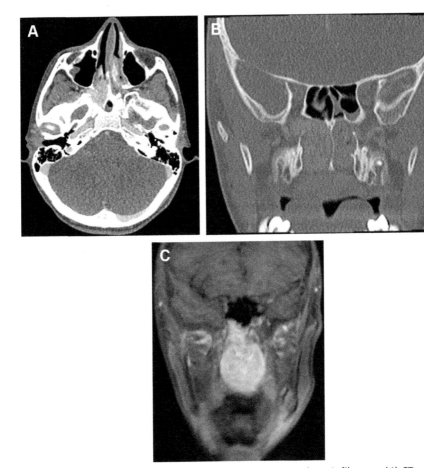

**Fig. 6.** CT and MRI demonstrating a juvenile nasopharyngeal angiofibroma. (*A*) CT axial. (*B*) CT coronal. (*C*) MRI T1 postcontrast coronal.

Alpha-fetoprotein has been used as a good marker for recurrence in the follow-up period but has limited utility as an initial diagnostic screening tool.[33]

### Malignant Nasal Masses

Although uncommon, there are many different types of malignant nasal masses that can present with nasal obstruction. These masses will usually present with other symptoms, such as change in smell, epistaxis, nasal/facial pain, or numbness in conjunction with the nasal obstruction. The nasal cavity mucosa is lined with minor salivary glands, which can lead to the development of salivary gland tumors (adenocarcinoma or adenoid cystic adenomas). Other types of malignant nasal masses that can present with nasal obstruction include rhabdomyosarcoma, esthesioneuroblastoma, lymphoma, squamous cell carcinoma, and metastatic disease.

Nasopharyngeal carcinoma (NPC) accounts for 20% to 50% of all primary childhood nasopharyngeal malignant tumors. It can present with nasal obstructive symptoms due to blockage of the posterior choanae. NPCs are frequently associated

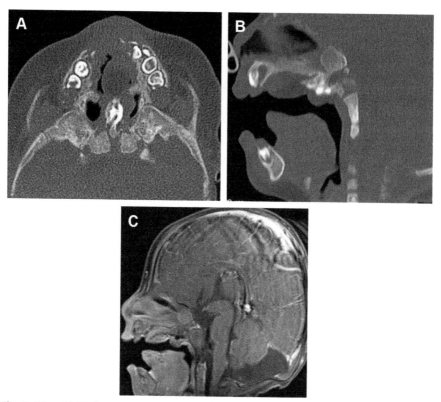

**Fig. 7.** CT and MRI demonstrating nasopharyngeal teratoma. (*A*) CT axial. (*B*) CT sagittal. (*C*) MRI T1 postcontrast sagittal.

with the Epstein-Barr virus, and titers are used for prognostication. Following nasal endoscopy, CT and MRI are both used for imaging this area and provide help with proper staging to assess the extent of local spread. Radiation is the standard treatment of early stage disease (1 and 2) and the addition of chemotherapy to the treatment regimen for late-stage disease (3 and 4).

## SUMMARY

Pediatric nasal obstruction is a common complaint, and the diagnosis and treatment of conditions causing this symptom varies. In infants and newborns, several congenital lesions may contribute to feeding and respiratory complaints. In older children, infectious causes, such as sinusitis and allergic rhinitis, are common and are treated medically, in a manner almost identical to adult treatment of these entities. Both trauma and neoplastic disease are alternative causes that can be diagnosed with nasal and/or nasopharyngeal endoscopy, proper history, and imaging.

## REFERENCES

1. Neskey D, Eloy JA, Casiano RR. Nasal, septal, and turbinate anatomy and embryology. Otolaryngol Clin North Am 2009;42(2):193–205.

2. Flake CG, Ferguson CF. Congenital choanal atresia in infants and children. Ann Otol Rhinol Laryngol 1964;73:458–73.
3. Deutsch E, Kaufman M, Eilon A. Transnasal endoscopic management of choanal atresia. Int J Pediatr Otorhinolaryngol 1997;40(1):19–26.
4. Josephson GD, Vickery CL, Giles WC, et al. Transnasal endoscopic repair of congenital choanal atresia: long-term results. Arch Otolaryngol Head Neck Surg 1998;124(5):537–40.
5. Stankiewicz JA. The endoscopic repair of choanal atresia. Otolaryngol Head Neck Surg 1990;103(6):931–7.
6. Keller JL, Kacker A. Choanal atresia, CHARGE association, and congenital nasal stenosis. Otolaryngol Clin North Am 2000;33:1343–51.
7. Strychowsky JE, Kawai K, Moritz E, et al. To stent or not to stent? A meta-analysis of endonasal congenital bilateral choanal atresia repair. Laryngoscope 2016; 126(1):218–27.
8. Willging JP. Transpalatal repair of choanal atresia. In: Potsic WP, Cotton RT, Handler SD, et al, editors. Surgical pediatric otolaryngology. New York: Thieme Medical Publishers; 2016. p. 193–215.
9. Brown O, Myer C, Manning S. Congenital nasal pyriform aperture stenosis. Laryngoscope 1989;99:86–91.
10. Tate JR, Sykes J. Congenital nasal pyriform aperture stenosis. Otolaryngol Clin North Am 2009;42:521–5.
11. Patel VA, Carr MM. Congenital nasal obstruction in infants: a retrospective study and literature review. Int J Pediatr Otorhinolaryngol 2017;99:78–84.
12. Wormald R, Hinton-Bayre A, Bumbak P, et al. Congenital nasal pyriform aperture stenosis 5.7 mm or less is associated with surgical intervention: a pooled case series. Int J Pediatr Otorhinolaryngol 2015;79(11):1802–5.
13. Sessions R. Nasal dermoid sinuses: new concepts and explanations. Laryngoscope 1982;92:1–19.
14. Zapata S, Kearns DB. Nasal dermoids. Curr Opin Otolaryngol Head Neck Surg 2006;14:406–11.
15. Gorenstein A, Kern EB, Facer GW, et al. Nasal gliomas. Arch Otolaryngol 1980; 106:536–40.
16. Moody MW, Chi DM, Mason JC, et al. Tornwaldt's cyst: Incidence and a case report. Ear Nose Throat J 2007;86(1):45.
17. Barham HP, Wudel JM, Enzenauer RW, et al. Congenital nasolacrimal duct cyst/ dacryocystocele: an argument for a genetic basis. Allergy Rhinol (Providence) 2012;3(1):e46–9.
18. Rahimov F, Jugessur A, Murray JC. Genetics of nonsyndromic orofacial clefts. Cleft Palate Craniofac J 2012;49(1):73–91.
19. Farzal Z, Walsh J, Lopes de Rezende Barbosa G, et al. Volumetric nasal cavity analysis in children with unilateral and bilateral cleft lip and palate. Laryngoscope 2016;126(6):1475–80.
20. Nathan RA, Meltzer EO, Selner JC, et al. Prevalence of allergic rhinitis in the United States. J Allergy Clin Immunol 1997;99:S808–14.
21. Mallol J, Crane J, von Mutius E, et al. The international study of asthma and allergies in childhood (ISAAC) phase three: a global synthesis. Allergol Immunopathol 2013;41:73–85.
22. Gentile D, Bartholow A, Valovirta E, et al. Current and future directions in pediatric allergic rhinitis. J Allergy Clin Immunol 2013;1:214–26.
23. Tharpe CA, Kemp SF. Pediatric allergic rhinitis. Immunol Allergy Clin North Am 2015;35(1):185–98.

24. Arganbright JM, Jensen EL, Mattingly J, et al. Utility of inferior turbinoplasty for the treatment of nasal obstruction in children: a 10-year review. JAMA Otolaryngol Head Neck Surg 2015;141(10):901–4.
25. Smart BA. The impact of allergic and nonallergic rhinitis on pediatric sinusitis. Curr Allergy Asthma Rep 2006;6:221–7.
26. Cunningham MJ, Chiu EJ, Landgraf JM, et al. The health impact of chronic recurrent rhinosinusitis in children. Arch Otolaryngol Head Neck Surg 2000;126: 1363–8.
27. Brietzke SE, Brigger MT. Adenoidectomy outcomes in pediatric rhinosinusitis: a meta-analysis. Int J Pediatr Otorhinolaryngol 2008;72(10):1541–5.
28. Ramadan HH, Cost JL. Outcome of adenoidectomy versus adenoidectomy with maxillary sinus wash for chronic rhinosinusitis in children. Laryngoscope 2008; 118(5):871–3.
29. Soler ZM, Rosenbloom JS, Skarada D, et al. Prospective, multicenter evaluation of balloon sinus dilation for treatment of pediatric chronic rhinosinusitis. Int Forum Allergy Rhinol 2017;7(3):221–9.
30. Haapaniemi JJ, Suonpää JT, Salmivalli AJ, et al. Prevalence of septal deviations in school-aged children. Rhinology 1995;33(1):1–3.
31. Reitzen SD, Chung W, Shah AR. Nasal septal deviation in the pediatric and adult populations. Ear Nose Throat J 2011;90(3):112–5.
32. Lawrence R. Pediatric septoplasty: a review of the literature. Int J Pediatr Otorhinolaryngol 2012;76(8):1078–81.
33. Alexander VR, Manjaly JG, Pepper CM, et al. Head and neck teratomas in children - a series of 23 cases at Great Ormond Street Hospital. Int J Pediatr Otorhinolaryngol 2015;79(12):2008–14.

# Nasal Obstruction Considerations in Cosmetic Rhinoplasty

Douglas Sidle, MD*, Katherine Hicks, MD, MS

## KEYWORDS

- Cosmetic rhinoplasty • Obstruction • Internal nasal valve • External nasal valve
- Surgical technique • Nasal valve compromise

## KEY POINTS

- During rhinoplasty, an aesthetically pleasing result may come at the expense of functional integrity if thorough preoperative examination and surgical planning have not been done.
- An intimate knowledge of nasal anatomy and physiology is critical in optimizing form and function during rhinoplasty.
- Successful rhinoplasty surgeons are adept at using strategies and techniques designed to prevent and/or ameliorate postoperative obstruction.
- The importance of counseling and establishing rapport with patients cannot be overstated.

## INTRODUCTION

Over the last 20 years, rhinoplasty has consistently been one of the most popular cosmetic surgeries in the United States, with more than 200,000 procedures performed annually.[1] However, often inherent in the pursuit of an aesthetically pleasing nose are structural changes that may compromise nasal patency, particularly with respect to narrowing of the internal nasal valve (INV) and external nasal valve (ENV) (**Fig. 1**). Previously existing anatomic or mucosal abnormalities render some patients particularly susceptible to obstruction postoperatively, and these patients require careful preoperative evaluation and surgical planning.

A previous study examining post-rhinoplasty nasal obstruction demonstrated a reduction in the cross-sectional area at the INV and pyriform aperture by 25% and 13%, respectively.[2] A different study estimated that 75% to 85% of patients have

Disclosures: D. Sidle is a speaker for and receives honoraria from Spirox Inc. K. Hicks has nothing to disclose.
Department of Otolaryngology–Head & Neck Surgery, McGaw Medical Center of Northwestern University, 676 North Saint Clair Street, Suite 1325, Chicago, IL 60611, USA
* Corresponding author.
E-mail address: Dsidle@nm.org

Otolaryngol Clin N Am 51 (2018) 987–1002
https://doi.org/10.1016/j.otc.2018.05.011
0030-6665/18/Published by Elsevier Inc.

oto.theclinics.com

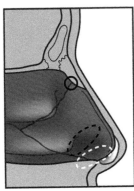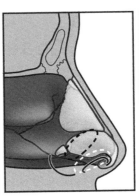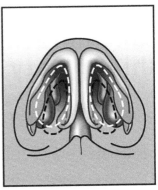

**Fig. 1.** The ENV (*white dashed line*), INV (*black dashed line*), and keystone region (*solid black line*). (*Courtesy of* Douglas Sidle, MD, Chicago, IL.)

some degree of narrowing at the nasal vestibule following rhinoplasty.[3] In keeping with these anatomic observations, it has been estimated that 10% of patients report subjective nasal obstruction following rhinoplasty,[4,5] and previous rhinoplasty has been shown to be the leading cause of obstruction prompting patients to seek nasal valve reconstruction.[6] Thus, during preoperative planning and intraoperative maneuvers, it is important to anticipate which maneuvers may negatively affect the static and dynamic support mechanisms critical to maintaining nasal airway patency and take preventative measures to avoid disrupting them.

## PERTINENT ANATOMY AND PHYSIOLOGY OF NASAL OBSTRUCTION

The prevention or repair of iatrogenic nasal obstruction begins with a thorough understanding of and appreciation for the intricate framework of the nose and the interplay among its bony, cartilaginous, and soft tissue components. Nasal patency is achieved when these components are structurally sound and do not result in obstruction at rest or with inhalation. Causes of inflammatory pathology of the nasal mucosa are myriad, and a thorough discussion is beyond the scope of this article; however, it is critical to identify and address any concomitant mucosal pathology before performing cosmetic or functional rhinoplasty.[7]

Defining nasal obstruction consists of localizing each contributing anatomic deformity and categorizing the problem as static, dynamic, or both. During analysis, it is helpful to divide the nose into vertical thirds and evaluate the structural components of each (**Fig. 2**).

The upper third of the nose, or bony vault, is comprised of paired nasal bones that articulate with the frontal bone superiorly and the ascending process of the maxilla laterally. They are thickest at their fusion with the frontal bone at the nasion and thinner caudally where they articulate with the upper lateral cartilages (ULC).[8] The keystone area (see **Fig. 1**) represents the region where the septum, perpendicular plate of the ethmoid, ULC, and nasal bones converge, and it is integral in supporting the nasal dorsum.[9]

The middle third, or cartilaginous vault, consists of the paired ULC, which are supported by fibrous connections to the caudal end of the nasal bones superiorly, the pyriform aperture laterally, and the dorsal septum medially. The INV complex as introduced by Mink in 1903 represents the cross-sectional area bounded by the dorsal septum, caudal end of the ULC, and head of the inferior turbinate.[10] The angle of the

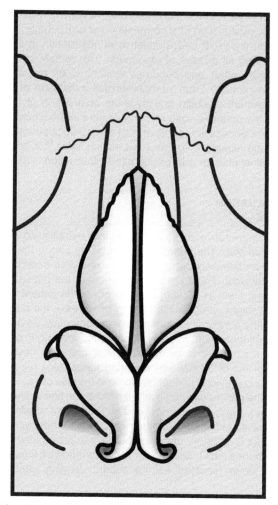

**Fig. 2.** It is helpful to divide the nose into vertical thirds: (1) bony vault, comprised of the nasal bones; (2) cartilaginous vault, comprised of the upper lateral cartilages and dorsal septum; and (3) tip region, comprised of the lower lateral cartilages and fibrofatty tissue. (*Courtesy of* Douglas Sidle, MD, Chicago, IL.)

valve should be between 10° and 15° in white noses and is slightly more obtuse in Asian and African noses.[11,12] Many maneuvers in cosmetic rhinoplasty place the integrity of this valve at risk, and preservation or augmentation of this angle during rhinoplasty is critical.

The lower third of the nose consists of the tip and alar structures, whose shape and strength are largely contingent on the composition and orientation of the lower lateral cartilages (LLC). The LLC are supported by fibrous attachments to the caudal septum, pyriform aperture, and ULC, and the relationship between the LLC and ULC in the scroll region is a major tip support mechanism.[8] The ENV represents the area bound by the caudal margin of the LLC, caudal septum, and soft tissue of the alar rim and nasal sill.[13] The approaches to and manipulation of the cartilages during tip work place the ENV at risk during cosmetic rhinoplasty.

Nasal obstruction in each of the aforementioned anatomic regions may be caused by static or dynamic dysfunction or a combination of both. Static dysfunction results from anatomic deformities that cause continuous obstruction at a specific region of the nasal airway during all phases of respiration. Conversely, dynamic dysfunction varies with respiratory effort and becomes evident when negative pressures are generated during inspiration. Thus, comprehensive evaluation of nasal obstruction must include assessment of static and dynamic obstruction at the upper, middle, and lower thirds of the patient's nose and should take into account a patient's native anatomy, and any evidence of iatrogenic or post-traumatic obstruction. Using an algorithm, such as the one recently presented by Lee and Most,[14] is helpful in developing an appropriate surgical plan for addressing nasal obstruction.

## PREOPERATIVE EVALUATION
### History and Physical

A comprehensive preoperative visit is paramount in establishing realistic goals and formulating a surgical plan. The consultation begins by asking the patient what specific aesthetic and functional concerns he or she has and proceeds with taking a thorough history and physical. There are a few aspects of the patient's history that are particularly important, such as eliciting whether or not the patient has any inflammatory conditions that might compromise healing or increase the risk of postoperative nasal obstruction. Any concomitant mucosal pathology must be optimally controlled before scheduling rhinoplasty. It is also critical to inquire about prior nasal surgery, because previous rhinoplasty is by far the most common cause of nasal valve dysfunction. In a review of 53 patients requiring nasal valve reconstruction, Khosh and colleagues[6] found previous rhinoplasty to be the cause of nasal valve obstruction in 79% of cases. If the patient has had surgery before, the timing and extent of surgery must be established, because scarring and deficiency of available cartilage may significantly alter the surgical plan. Another important element of a patient's history is determining if there is a history of nasal trauma, because it may result in displacement of the nasal bones, ULC, septum, or a combination of these structures. Prior nasal trauma has been reported as the second leading cause of nasal valve dysfunction.[15]

The physical examination entails assessment of the external appearance of the nose and visualization of the nasal cavity. It is important to have a systematic method for assessing the external appearance of the nose and to make note of features that may be responsible for existing obstruction or may predispose a patient to post-rhinoplasty obstruction. The nose should be evaluated from profile, frontal, and basal views, and standardized, representative photographs should be taken and stored for documentation. A recent consensus statement supports consideration of photography, because it may be useful in documenting external deformities commonly associated with nasal valve collapse.[16] In our practice, we routinely use preoperative computer imaging ("morphed" images) to facilitate communication with the patient regarding postoperative expectations. Recent studies report that computer imaging is viewed favorably by patients and is at least moderately accurate in predicting postoperative outcomes.[17–19]

Internally, anterior rhinoscopy generally allows for examination of the caudal septum, inferior turbinates, and general condition of the nasal mucosa. However, performing only anterior rhinoscopy may overlook concomitant problems that could be addressed at the time of surgery, and endoscopic evaluation should be considered when applicable. Recently, it has been reported that between 29% and 39% of patients had findings on nasal endoscopy that were not visible on anterior rhinoscopy and ultimately required additional surgical management, including sinus surgery, concha bullosa resection, posterior endoscopic septoplasty, or adenoidectomy; in one case, an intranasal tumor was identified via nasal endoscopy.[20,21] Similarly, a recent clinical consensus statement reported that endoscopy could be useful in diagnosing collapse and ruling out other intranasal pathology.[16] These reports indicate that using nasal endoscopy during initial evaluation may help streamline and optimize treatment.[20,21] For anterior rhinoscopy and nasal endoscopy, evaluation of the nasal cavity before and after administration of topical decongestant is important.

One important aspect of the preoperative examination that must be emphasized is performance of the modified Cottle maneuver to identify nasal valve collapse.[22] This involves using an ear curette or similar instrument to support the ULC and then the LLC during inspiration to assess for dysfunction of the INV and ENV, respectively. When performing the maneuver, the valves should be supported, not lateralized to give a realistic assessment of improvement. This is done before and after application of topical decongestant. During each maneuver, the patient rates his or her nasal patency on a visual analog scale ranging from 0 (no patency) to 10 (maximum patency). Constantinides and colleagues[22] reported that this maneuver was helpful in localizing obstruction and planning surgical intervention; in their study, 18 of 19 patients (94.7%) reported improved breathing following surgery when the Cottle maneuver was used to guide surgical decision-making. More recently, it has been reported that patients with a positive Cottle maneuver have 20% greater symptom burden at presentation and 24% less improvement after septoplasty and turbinate reduction when compared with patients undergoing the same procedure with a negative Cottle preoperatively.[23]

When performing the modified Cottle maneuver or visualizing the nasal cavity via anterior rhinoscopy or nasal endoscopy, it is common practice to evaluate before and after administration of topical decongestant to determine whether mucosal inflammation plays a significant role in a patient's nasal obstruction. If a patient experiences substantial improvement in nasal patency following administration of decongestant, inflammation likely plays a role in existing nasal obstruction, and the patient must be counseled that continued medical management will likely be necessary postoperatively.

Finally, all rhinoplasty surgeons should be aware of the body dysmorphic disorder patient. These patients often are critical of prior surgeons or of their perceived deformities. Likewise, they are overly fixated on their nose and the sensation of breathing. These patients may not be good candidates for a surgery where success is subjective.

### Notable Preoperative Findings

There are several pertinent findings on examination that may localize sources of current nasal obstruction or highlight areas that are at increased risk for obstruction following rhinoplasty. Although there is some anatomic and functional overlap between areas of the nose, it may be helpful to systematically evaluate the following anatomic areas to delineate current or potential sources of obstruction: (1) INV, (2) ENV, and (3) other intranasal deformity. It is important to carefully document these findings, discuss them with patients, and take them into account when developing a surgical plan.

### Internal nasal valve

Most obstruction in the upper and middle thirds of the nose is related to static deformity or dynamic dysfunction of components of the INV, the angle of which generally measures at least 10° to 15° (**Fig. 3**). Thus, deviation or weakness of the septum,

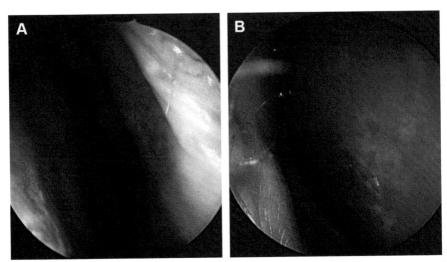

**Fig. 3.** (*A*) Normal internal nasal valve angle of 10° to 15°. (*B*) Abnormally narrow internal nasal valve. (*Courtesy of* Douglas Sidle, MD, Chicago, IL.)

hypertrophy or medialization of the inferior turbinates, and destabilization or collapse of the ULC in this region all contribute to nasal obstruction in this area.

Patients with short nasal bones, narrow middle vault, weak ULC, thin skin, or a combination of these factors are predisposed to INV collapse.[3] Short nasal bones are at increased risk of fragmentation during osteotomies, and they are associated with long ULC that render the middle vault prone to collapse.[24] The characteristic inverted-V deformity shown in **Fig. 4**A, first described by Sheen,[3] indicates the presence of middle vault collapse and should be addressed for cosmetic and functional purposes. Patients with facial weakness or paralysis are also at increased risk for INV compromise, because dysfunction of the nasal muscles,[25] particularly dilator nasalis and nasalis transversalis,[26] has been seen in patients with dynamic valve collapse. A patient's age must be taken into account, because aging may weaken the connective tissue of the nasal sidewall, rendering it prone to collapse with inspiration.[27]

*External nasal valve*
Most obstruction in the lower third of the nose is related to static deformity or dynamic dysfunction of components of the ENV. Thus, primary causes of obstruction at this level include deformity of the caudal septum, LLC deficiency or malposition, and weakness or stenosis of the soft tissues of the alar rim and nasal sill.

Although most patients with INV dysfunction present with a history of trauma or previous rhinoplasty, ENV collapse is frequently seen in patients who have not had previous nasal surgery.[28] From a basal view, patients with ENV frequently have narrow, slit-like nostrils (**Fig. 4**C) that exhibit alar collapse with inspiration. Factors that contribute to this nostril configuration include the following: wide columella, narrow alar base, overly projected tip, thin alar sidewalls, and weak or malpositioned LLC.[3,28] Significant recurvature (**Fig. 4**D) of the LLC should also alert the physician to the presence of or propensity for ENV compromise. The parenthesis deformity, first described by Sheen,[29] denotes cephalic malpositioning of the LLC, which manifests as a boxy tip with notching of the alar rim. In other patients, tip ptosis attributable to myriad causes may exacerbate ENV collapse. Finally, patients with

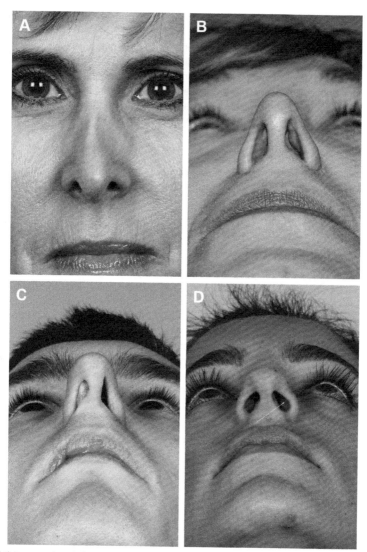

**Fig. 4.** (*A*) Inverted-V deformity with prominent collapse of ULC. (*B*) Significantly compromised, narrow INV. (*C*) Severe caudal septal deviation and slit-like nostrils with compromise of ENV. (*D*) Strong recurvature of the lateral crus of the LLC (*white arrow*). (*Courtesy of Douglas Sidle, MD, Chicago, IL.*)

a history of burns or inhalation injury, previous cutaneous neoplasm, or poorly executed rim or marginal incisions are at risk of tissue loss, scarring, and vestibular stenosis.

## Other intranasal obstruction

Nasal septal deviations are often a result of previous trauma and may result in clinically significant obstruction. It is important to visualize all portions of the septum that are likely contributing to obstruction, which may require nasal endoscopy. Even in the absence of deviations or spurs, weakened septal cartilage caused by inflammatory processes, such as granulomatosis with polyangiitis, may compromise the integrity of the nasal framework.

The head of the inferior turbinate represents one boundary of the INV, and hypertrophy of the inferior turbinate may result in clinically significant nasal obstruction. Other potential intranasal sources of obstruction include mucosal inflammation, nasal polyposis, concha bullosa of the middle turbinate, and mass within the nasal cavity or paranasal sinuses. A thorough preoperative evaluation including the components listed in **Box 1** is necessary to avoid neglecting any source of obstruction during surgery.

## INTRAOPERATIVE CONSIDERATIONS

Previous rhinoplasty is the most common cause of nasal valve dysfunction,[6] and primary rhinoplasty may result in clinically significant obstruction if meticulous technique and prophylactic measures are not used during surgery. Within each area of the nose, care must be taken to relieve existing obstruction, preserve structural support, and address any factors that would predispose a patient to postoperative obstruction.

### Internal Nasal Valve

Maneuvers that may compromise the integrity of the INV usually involve manipulation of the nasal bones, ULC, or dorsal septum. It is important to maintain or augment the structural support and angle of the INV.

Osteotomies are often performed during cosmetic rhinoplasty to straighten or narrow the nasal dorsum or to close an open roof deformity following dorsal hump reduction. However, improperly performed osteotomies result in instability of the upper and middle vaults and subsequent constriction of the INV.[30] When performing osteotomies, conservative elevation of periosteum with preservation of a soft tissue envelope is important.[31–33] It is generally considered safe to perform lateral osteotomies in a

---

**Box 1**
**Key components of prerhinoplasty history and physical**

*History*

Previous nasal surgery

Previous trauma

Medications, prescription and over-the-counter

Presence of localized inflammatory disorder (eg, chronic rhinosinusitis)

Presence of systemic inflammatory disorder (allergic/immunologic)

*Physical*

Visualize
  Skin quality and thickness
  Presence of external deformity (eg, inverted-V, parenthesis)
  Nasal cavity (anterior rhinoscopy, nasal endoscopy if indicated)

Palpate
  Length of nasal bones
  Strength and position of alar cartilages
  Position and length of the caudal septum

Perform
  Modified Cottle maneuver
  Oxymetazoline challenge
  Consider nasal endoscopy

high-low-high pathway, initiating the osteotomy a few millimeters above the head of the inferior turbinate. This technique preserves the integrity of the lateral suspensory ligaments and prevents medialization of the inferior turbinates and ULC.[34,35]

During dorsal hump reduction, the ULC are often separated from the dorsal septum, and overly aggressive osteotomy approaches may rarely result in disruption of the ULC attachment to the nasal bones. Adequate resuspension and support of the ULC is critical to maintaining the integrity of the INV. This is commonly achieved via placement of a spreader graft (**Fig. 5**), which entails harvesting a long, thin cartilage graft from the septum and inserting it between the dorsal septum and medial aspect of the ULC. This augments the INV area and is intended to prevent development of an inverted-V or hourglass deformity. Since its introduction by Sheen in 1984,[3] there have been several variations described in the literature, including endonasal placement,[36,37] use of polymeric implants when autologous tissue is unavailable,[38] and medial infolding of a narrow strip of ULC as an "autospreader" or "spreader flap."[39,40]

Another frequently used method of supporting the ULC that may be used in conjunction with spreader grafts is placement of a flaring suture, which was introduced by Park[41] in 1998 and found to subjectively improve nasal patency in all patients included in his initial study. A subsequent cadaver study showed an increase in the minimum cross-sectional area at the INV following placement of spreader grafts (5.4%), flaring sutures (9.1%), or both; the largest increase (18.7%) was seen when both methods were used.[42] Other groups have advocated slightly different strategies, wherein the medial aspect of the ULCs are mobilized and suspended over the nasal dorsum with[43] or without[44] the placement of underlying dorsal grafts.

Finally, meticulous placement and closure of incisions are essential in avoiding stenosis in the INV. Intercartilaginous incisions are located in the scroll region, at the junction of the LLC and ULC. When these incisions are poorly placed or improperly reapproximated, mucosal stenosis may occur, and the scroll area may be destabilized.[45]

### External Nasal Valve

Maneuvers that may compromise the integrity of the ENV usually involve manipulation of the LLC but may also be seen with manipulation of the caudal septum or narrowing of the alar base.

Probably the most commonly cited error in the lower third of the nose is overresection of the LLC when performing a cephalic trim. If one is to be performed, leaving a

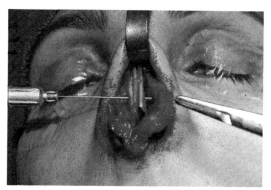

**Fig. 5.** Placement of spreader grafts to augment and support the internal nasal valve. (*Courtesy of* Douglas Sidle, MD, Chicago, IL.)

residual strip of at least 5 to 7 mm is generally recommended to prevent ENV collapse, alar retraction, and formation of bossae.[46,47] A recent study used animal and computer models to evaluate the strength of the LLC and found a decrease in mechanical stability in struts less than 6 mm.[48]

To avoid cartilage deficiency and loss of strength, attention has shifted toward efforts to conserve cartilage while also achieving a cosmetically acceptable tip. Several authors advocate cephalic turn-in flaps (**Fig. 6**), wherein the strip of cartilage that would have been removed during a cephalic trim is instead left attached on its deep surface and then folded underneath the remaining lateral crus. Introduced in 2007,[49] this technique achieves the same cosmetic result while maintaining or increasing the strength of the LLC.[50,51] The lateral crural steal maneuver is an alternative technique that repositions the lateral crura medially to increase tip projection and rotation while maintaining the stability of the alar cartilage complex.[52] Performing a lateral crural steal in combination with a septal extension graft has been termed lateral

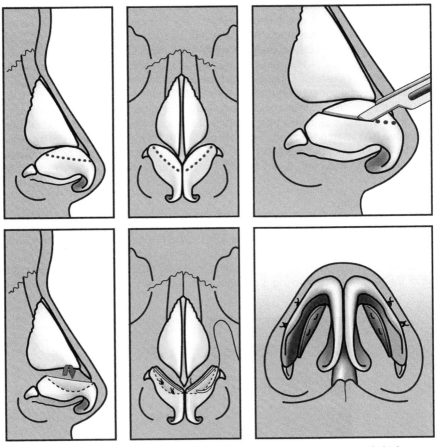

**Fig. 6.** Cephalic turn-in flaps used to stabilize the nasal valve region. A partial-thickness cut is made to the cephalic portion of the lower lateral cartilage using a #15 blade, extending down to the perichondrium on the deep surface of the cartilage. This strip is then folded under the remainder of the cartilage and secured with a polypropylene suture. This achieves improved tip contour while maintaining support of the nasal valve. (*Courtesy of* Douglas Sidle, MD, Chicago, IL.)

crural tensioning, and this has enhanced the strength and versatility of this technique.[53,54]

There is a multitude of different suture techniques used to refine tip projection, rotation, and contour.[55] However, these must be used judiciously to prevent overnarrowing of the nasal airway. In particular, overly aggressive transdomal or interdomal sutures may increase recurvature of the lateral crura and compromise nasal patency.

Alar rim retraction and alar collapse are problematic from a functional and cosmetic standpoint. Alar rim grafting (**Fig. 7**) entails insertion of a thin cartilage graft in a slim soft tissue pocket created just above the alar rim[56,57]; some authors have advocated suturing these grafts to the underlying tip complex to further enhance stability.[58] These grafts are designed to improve the integrity of the ENV and prevent or correct alar notching.

### Septum and Inferior Turbinates

Janki Shah and colleagues' article, "Techniques in Septoplasty: Traditional Versus Endoscopic Approaches," and Regan W. Bergmark and Stacey T. Gray's article, "Surgical Management of Turbinate Hypertrophy," in this issue, are devoted to management of the septum and inferior turbinates, respectively, so the following represents just a few key points that the author believes are particularly important during cosmetic rhinoplasty. Addressing all clinically significant septal deviations while maintaining the strength and integrity of the nasal framework is essential. Whether correcting deviations, harvesting grafts, or both, it has been shown that leaving an L-strut of 10 to 15 mm or greater is required to maintain stability and prevent the development of saddle nose deformity.[59,60] A technique favored by this author for graft harvest is to use the posteroinferior portion of the quadrangular cartilage and bevel the posterosuperior cut as shown in **Fig. 8**. Anecdotally, this has increased stability and prevented bowing of the septum at this critical area.

With respect to inferior turbinate reduction, there are many different techniques used by rhinologists and facial plastic surgeons. Some of the most commonly used methods include submucous resection,[61] microdebrider reduction,[62] outfracture of the turbinate,[63] radiofrequency ablation,[64] and submucous coblation.[62] In general, there is a lack of consensus in the literature regarding which technique is most effective. A recent systematic review of 96 articles describing outcomes after inferior

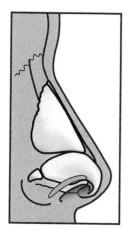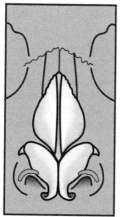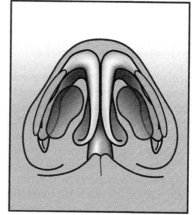

**Fig. 7.** Alar rim grafts to stabilize the external nasal valve. (*Courtesy of* Douglas Sidle, MD, Chicago, IL.)

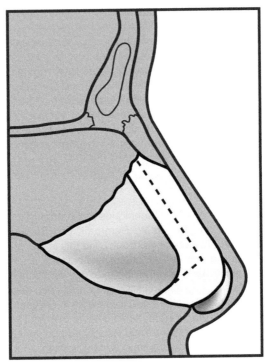

**Fig. 8.** When performing septoplasty and/or harvesting septal cartilage, it is prudent to maintain a stable connection between the dorsal and caudal struts. Traditionally, an L-strut is left at the dorsal and caudal aspects of the septal cartilage (*dashed line*). The senior author prefers to use a more conservative beveled cut near the anterior septal angle to avoid buckling of the quadrangular cartilage at this weak point. (*Courtesy of* Douglas Sidle, MD, Chicago, IL.)

turbinate reduction demonstrated significant improvement in subjective and objective measures following surgery, regardless of technique.[65] It is the senior author's common practice to, at minimum, cauterize the turbinates, outfracture them, and apply Doyle splints after septoplasty to help keep the turbinates lateralized. None of this has any cost to our cosmetic patients.

## POSTOPERATIVE MANAGEMENT

Perhaps the most important aspect of postoperative management is a thorough preoperative discussion about expectations. Patients should be prepared for swelling and ecchymosis following surgery and should know that in some cases, edema may take many months to completely resolve. Thus, during the initial postoperative period, providing reassurance is essential. In the absence of a glaring technical error that would best be served with early intervention, we recommend waiting at least 6 months before considering any type of revision.

If a patient complains of nasal obstruction postoperatively, one could first offer intranasal topical steroids or other medical management. Patients who continue to complain of obstruction more than 6 months after surgery may require additional management beyond medical therapy. A thorough investigation into the cause of nasal obstruction, including evaluation of the posterior nasal cavity and nasopharynx if not done preoperatively, is essential. One noninvasive option that may be considered if valve collapse is suspected is insertion of an absorbable nasal implant. A recent study evaluating nasal obstruction in 30 patients before and after insertion of the Latera device (Spirox Inc, Redwood City, CA) reported a mean reduction in the NOSE score of 40.9 points and no negative cosmetic effects 12 months after insertion.[66]

## SUMMARY

Preoperative and postoperative communication with patients undergoing cosmetic rhinoplasty is essential. The surgeon must fully understand the goals of each patient, and each patient must have appropriate short- and long-term expectations following surgery. From preoperative planning to surgery to postoperative care, thoughtful consideration must be given to correcting existing nasal obstruction and preventing iatrogenic obstruction following rhinoplasty.

## REFERENCES

1. American Society of Plastic Surgeons. 2016 Plastic Surgery Statistics Report. 2016. Available at: http://scholar.google.com/scholar?hl=en&btnG=Search&q=intitle: Plastic+Surgery+Statistics+Report#1. Accessed December 17, 2017.
2. Grymer L. Reduction rhinoplasty and nasal patency: change in the cross-sectional area of the nose evaluated by acoustic rhinometry. Laryngoscope 1995;105:429–31.
3. Sheen J. Spreader graft: a method of reconstructing the roof of the middle nasal vault following rhinoplasty. Plast Reconstr Surg 1984;73:230–7.
4. Beekhuis G. Nasal obstruction after rhinoplasty: etiology, and techniques for correction. Laryngoscope 1976;86:540–8.
5. Courtiss E, Goldwyn R. The effects of nasal surgery on airflow. Plast Reconstr Surg 1983;72:9–21.
6. Khosh M, Jen A, Honrado C, et al. Nasal valve reconstruction: experience in 53 consecutive patients. Arch Facial Plast Surg 2004;6(3):167–71.
7. Chandra RK, Patadia MO, Raviv J. Diagnosis of nasal airway obstruction. Otolaryngol Clin North Am 2009;42(2):207–25.
8. Tardy M. Surgical anatomy of the nose. New York: Raven Press; 1990.
9. Simon P, Lam K, Sidle D, et al. The nasal keystone region: an anatomical study. JAMA Facial Plast Surg 2013;15(3):235–7.
10. Mink PJ. Le nez comme voie respiratorie. Presse Otolaryngol 1903;21:481–96.
11. Kasperbauer JL, Kern E. Nasal valve physiology: implications in nasal surgery. Otolaryngol Clin North Am 1987;20:699–719.
12. Kern EB, Wang T. Nasal valve surgery. In: Daniel RK, Regnault P, Goldwyn R, editors. Aesthetic plastic surgery: rhinoplasty. Boston (MA): Little, Brown and Co; 1993. p. 613–30.
13. Constantian M. The incompetent external nasal valve: pathophysiology and treatment in primary and secondary rhinoplasty. Plast Reconstr Surg 1994; 93:919–31.
14. Lee MK, Most SP. Evidence-based medicine: rhinoplasty. Facial Plast Surg Clin North Am 2015;23(3):303–12.
15. Elwany S, Thabet H. Obstruction of the nasal valve. J Laryngol Otol 1996;100: 221–4.
16. Rhee JS, Weaver EM, Park SS, et al. Clinical consensus statement: diagnosis and management of nasal valve compromise. Otolaryngol Head Neck Surg 2010; 143(1):48–59.

17. Mehta U, Mazhar K, Frankel A. Accuracy of preoperative computer imaging in rhinoplasty. Arch Facial Plast Surg 2010;12(6):394–8.
18. Sharp H, Tingay R, Coman S, et al. Computer imaging and patient satisfaction in rhinoplasty surgery. J Laryngol Otol 2002;116(12):1009–13.
19. Muhlbauer W, Holm C. Computer imaging and surgical reality in aesthetic rhinoplasty. Plast Reconstr Surg 2005;115(7):2098–104.
20. Lanfranchi PV, Steiger J, Sparano A, et al. Diagnostic and surgical endoscopy in functional septorhinoplasty. Facial Plast Surg 2004;20(3):207–15.
21. Levine H. The office diagnosis of nasal and sinus disorders using rigid nasal endoscopy. Otolaryngol Head Neck Surg 1990;102:370–3.
22. Constantinides M, Galli S, Miller P. A simple and reliable method of patient evaluation in the surgical treatment of nasal obstruction. Ear Nose Throat J 2002; 81(10):734–7.
23. Bonaparte J, Cheung L. Does the Cottle maneuver predict outcomes after septal surgery? American Academy of Otolaryngology Head & Neck Surgery Annual Meeting. Dallas (TX), September 27-30, 2015.
24. Steele NP, Thomas J. Surgical anatomy of the nose. In: Stucker FJ, de Souza C, Kenyon GS, et al, editors. Rhinology and facial plastic surgery. New York: Springer Publishing; 2009. p. 5–12. https://doi.org/10.1016/S0030-6665(05)70119-5.
25. Kienstra MA, Gassner HG, Sherris DA, et al. Effects of the nasal muscles on the nasal airway. Am J Rhinol 2005;19:375–81.
26. Aksoy F, Veyseller B, Yildirim YS, et al. Role of nasal muscles in nasal valve collapse. Otolaryngol Head Neck Surg 2010;142(3):365–9.
27. Wittkopf M, Wittkopf J, Ries WR. The diagnosis and treatment of nasal valve collapse. Curr Opin Otolaryngol Head Neck Surg 2008;16(1):10–3.
28. Toriumi DM, Josen J, Weinberger M, et al. Use of alar batten grafts for correction of nasal valve collapse. Arch Otolaryngol Head Neck Surg 1997;123:802–8.
29. Sheen J. Aesthetic rhinoplasty. Maryland Heights (MO): Mosby, Inc; 1978. p. 264–5.
30. Guyuron B. Nasal osteotomy and airway changes. Plast Reconstr Surg 1998;102: 856–60.
31. Farrior R. The osteotomy in rhinoplasty. Laryngoscope 1978;88:1449–59.
32. Thomas JR, Griner NR, Remmler DJ. Steps for a safer method of osteotomies in rhinoplasty. Laryngoscope 1987;97(6):746–7.
33. Webster RC, Davidson TM, Smith R. Curved lateral osteotomy for airway protection in rhinoplasty. Arch Otolaryngol Head Neck Surg 1977;103:454–8.
34. Most SP, Murakami CS. Nasal osteotomies: anatomy, planning, and technique. Facial Plast Surg Clin North Am 2002;10(3):279–85.
35. Anderson J. A new approach to rhinoplasty. Trans Am Acad Ophthalmol Otolaryngol 1966;70:183–92.
36. André RF, Paun SH, Vuyk HD. Endonasal spreader graft placement as treatment for internal nasal valve insufficiency: no need to divide the upper lateral cartilages from the septum. Arch Facial Plast Surg 2004;6(1):36–40.
37. Yoo D, Jen A. Endonasal placement of spreader grafts: experience in 41 consecutive patients. Arch Facial Plast Surg 2012;14:318–22.
38. Reiffel AJ, Cross KJ, Spinelli HM. Nasal spreader grafts: a comparison of Medpor to autologous tissue reconstruction. Ann Plast Surg 2011;66(1):24–8.
39. Byrd HS, Meade RA, Gonyon DL. Using thed. Plast Reconstr Surg 2007;119(6): 1897–902.
40. Gruber RP, Park E, Newman J, et al. The spreader flap in primary rhinoplasty. Plast Reconstr Surg 2007;119(6):1903–10.

41. Park S. The flaring suture to augment the repair of the dysfunctional nasal valve. Plast Reconstr Surg 1998;101:1120–2.
42. Schlosser RJ, Park SS. Surgery for the dysfunctional nasal valve. Arch Facial Plast Surg 1999;1:105–10.
43. Sciuto S, Bernardeschi D. Upper lateral cartilage suspension over dorsal grafts: a treatment for internal nasal valve dynamic incompetence. Facial Plast Surg 1999; 15(4):309–16.
44. Fayman MS, Potgieter E. Nasal middle vault support: a new technique. Aesthetic Plast Surg 2004;28(6):375–80.
45. Adamson J. Constriction of the internal nasal valve in rhinoplasty: treatment and prevention. Ann Plast Surg 1987;18:114–21.
46. Gubisch W, Eichhorn-Sens J. Overresection of the lower lateral cartilages: a common conceptual mistake with functional and aesthetic consequences. Aesthetic Plast Surg 2009;33(1):6–13.
47. Pedroza F, Anjos G, Patrocinio L, et al. Seagull wing graft: a technique for the replacement of the lower lateral cartilages. Arch Facial Plast Surg 2006;8(6):396–403.
48. Oliaei S, Manuel C, Protsenko D, et al. Mechanical analysis of the effects of cephalic trim on lower lateral cartilage stability. Arch Facial Plast Surg 2012;14(1):27–30.
49. Tellioglu AT, Cimen K. Turn-in folding of the cephalic portion of the lateral crus to support the alar rim in rhinoplasty. Aesthetic Plast Surg 2007;31(3):306–10.
50. Barham HP, Knisely A, Christensen J, et al. Costal cartilage lateral crural strut graft vs cephalic crural turn-in for correction of external valve dysfunction. JAMA Facial Plast Surg 2015;17(5):340.
51. Murakami CS, Barrera JE, Most SP. Preserving structural integrity of the alar cartilage in aesthetic rhinoplasty using a cephalic turn-in flap. Arch Facial Plast Surg 2009;11(2):126–8.
52. Kridel R, Konior R, Shumrick K, et al. Advances in nasal tip surgery: the lateral crural steal. Arch Otolaryngol Head Neck Surg 1989;115:1206–12.
53. Davis RE. Lateral crural tensioning for refinement of the wide and underprojected nasal tip: rethinking the lateral crural steal. Facial Plast Surg Clin North Am 2015; 23:23–53.
54. Davis R. Revision of the over-resected tip/alar cartilage complex. Facial Plast Surg 2012;28(4):427–39.
55. Cingi C, Muluk N, Ulusoy S, et al. Nasal tip sutures: techniques and indications. Am J Rhinol Allergy 2015;29(6):205–11.
56. Rohrich RJ, Raniere J Jr, Ha R. The alar contour graft: correction and prevention of alar rim deformities in rhinoplasty. Plast Reconstr Surg 2002;109:2495–505.
57. Troell RJ, Powell NB, Riley RW, et al. Evaluation of a new procedure for nasal alar rim and valve collapse: nasal alar rim reconstruction. Otolaryngol Head Neck Surg 2000;122(2):204–11.
58. Ballin AC, Kim H, Chance E, et al. The articulated alar rim graft: reengineering the conventional alar rim graft for improved contour and support. Facial Plast Surg 2016;32(4):384–97.
59. Killian G. The submucous window resection of the nasal septum. Ann Otol Rhinol Laryngol 1905;14:363–93.
60. Mau T, Mau S, Kim D. Cadaveric and engineering analysis of the septal L-strut. Laryngoscope 2007;117(11):1902–6.
61. Spielberg W. The treatment of nasal obstruction by submucous resection of the inferior turbinate bone. Laryngoscope 1924;34:197–203.
62. Hegazy H, ElBadawey M, Behery A. Inferior turbinate reduction; coblation versus microdebrider - a prospective, randomised study. Rhinology 2014;52(4):306–14.

63. Aksoy F, Yildirim Y, Veyseller B, et al. Midterm outcomes of outfracture of the inferior turbinate. Otolaryngol Head Neck Surg 2010;143(4):579–84.
64. Harrill W, Pillsbury H. Radiofrequency turbinate reduction: a NOSE evaluation. Laryngoscope 2007;117(11):1912–9.
65. Batra P, Seiden A, Smith T. Surgical management of adult inferior turbinate hypertrophy: a systematic review of the evidence. Laryngoscope 2009;119(9): 1819–27.
66. San Nicolo M, Stelter K, Sadick H, et al. Absorbable implant to treat nasal valve collapse. Facial Plast Surg 2017;32:233–40.

# Nasal Obstruction Considerations in Sleep Apnea

Mahmoud I. Awad, MD, Ashutosh Kacker, MD*

## KEYWORDS

- Nasal obstruction • Obstructive sleep apnea • Sleep-disordered breathing
- Nasal surgery • Septoplasty • Turbinate reduction

## KEY POINTS

- The nasal airway plays a significant role in breathing during sleep and, therefore, nasal obstruction can result in sleep-disordered breathing.
- Topical nasal steroids can improve sleep quality, but the evidence for their role in the treatment of obstructive sleep apnea (OSA) is not as strong.
- Surgery to correct nasal obstruction has similarly been shown to improve sleep quality but not necessarily sleep apnea.
- Nasal obstruction surgery may facilitate treatment of patients with OSA by improving tolerance and compliance with continuous positive airway pressure.

## INTRODUCTION

Obstructive sleep apnea (OSA), characterized by recurrent episodes of upper airway obstructing occurring during sleep, is a very prevalent condition.[1] According to the Wisconsin Sleep Cohort Study, published in 1993, an estimated 9% of women and 24% of men aged 30 to 60 years have this condition in the United States alone.[2] Given the association between weight gain and obesity and OSA,[3] these data were recently reexamined in the context of the global obesity epidemic, and prevalence estimates increased to 17% and 34%, respectively.[4]

Left untreated, the condition is associated with an increased risk for cardiovascular disease. In addition to representing a significant risk factor for hypertension, coronary artery disease, and stroke,[5-7] OSA is associated with an increased risk of diabetes and cancer.[8,9] It also has significant psychosocial implications, impacting cognitive

Disclosure: The authors have nothing to disclose.
Department of Otolaryngology–Head and Neck Surgery, Weill Cornell Medical College, 1305 York Avenue, 5th Floor, New York, NY 10021, USA
* Corresponding author. 1305 York Avenue, 5th Floor, New York, NY 10021.
E-mail address: ask9001@med.cornell.edu

Otolaryngol Clin N Am 51 (2018) 1003–1009
https://doi.org/10.1016/j.otc.2018.05.012
0030-6665/18/© 2018 Elsevier Inc. All rights reserved.

function, social interactions, and quality of life (QOL).[10] For these reasons, OSA has emerged to become a significant public health challenge globally.

The first-line treatment of OSA is continuous positive airway pressure (CPAP), which has been shown to reduce the risks of the aforementioned complications, improve QOL, and lower the rates of motor vehicle accidents.[11] Variable compliance to therapy, however, limits its overall effectiveness; 46% to 83% of patients are nonadherent.[12] The mask interface, discomfort from the air pressure required, nasal obstruction and dryness, and psychological and social factors lead to poor acceptance and nonadherence.[13] Although other nonsurgical treatment options exist, such as oral appliances, surgery may play a role in the treatment of this condition.

The severity of sleep apnea is usually assessed by the apnea-hypopnea index (AHI), which is defined as the average number of complete (apnea) and incomplete (hypopnea) obstructive events in 1 hour of sleep. In general, OSA is defined as an AHI of 5 or greater. Five to 14 is defined as mild disease, 15 to 29 as moderate disease, and 30 or greater as severe disease.[14] In general, a 50% reduction in AHI and a final AHI of 20 per hour or less is defined a surgical cure.[15]

## NASAL OBSTRUCTION AND SLEEP APNEA

Nasal obstruction is a known risk factor for sleep-disordered breathing secondary to changes in airflow velocity and resistance.[16] As the nose represents the first portal of air entry, nasal pathologic conditions in the form of septal deviation, nasal polyps, turbinate hypertrophy, and rhinitis can contribute to OSA.[17] Moreover, the nose accounts for 50% of the total upper airway resistance; serves many important physiologic functions, including humidification and filtration; and is the preferred breathing route during sleep.[18] In fact, the oral fraction of inhaled ventilation during sleep in healthy subjects with normal nasal resistance is only approximately 4%.[19]

Many pathophysiologic mechanisms have been described to explain the effect on nasal obstruction on sleep-disordered breathing. According to the Starling resistor model, apnea can occur when nasal obstruction generates enough negative intraluminal pressure downstream to cause the compliant soft tissues of the oropharynx to collapse.[20] In the face of significant nasal resistance, a compensatory switch to mouth breathing may occur. Oral breathing in sleep is physiologically unfavorable and unstable, however, and is associated with up to 2.5 times higher resistance secondary to narrowing of the pharyngeal lumen and further posterior collapse of the tongue, resulting in more frequent apneic events.[21] In addition, bypassing the nasal airway leads to less activation of nasal receptors and the nasal-ventilatory reflex, resulting in decreased muscle tone and ventilation secondary to decreased activation of nasal receptors.[22] Finally, significant nitric oxide production occurs in the nose. With mouth breathing, the decreased nitric oxide production leads to changes in the maintenance of muscle tone and changes in spontaneous ventilation and sleep patterns.[23]

There exists a body of clinical and experimental evidence that demonstrates an association between reducing nasal patency and sleep-disordered breathing. Patients with nasal packing experience decreased sleep quality and an increase in frequency of apneic episodes.[24] This finding was demonstrated in patients who undergo nasal packing for epistaxis[25] as well as in patients with packing after septoplasty.[26] Turhan and colleagues[27] specifically demonstrated significantly higher AHI scores and oxygen desaturations in patients treated with nasal packing compared with transseptal suture after septoplasty. Similar to artificially induced nasal obstruction, patients with chronic nasal congestion report sleep-disordered breathing.[28] Several studies have also demonstrated an association between seasonal allergic rhinitis and decreased sleep quality and an increase in apneic episodes.[29,30] In one study, patients with nonallergic rhinitis were at greater risk for higher AHI and Epworth Sleepiness Scale scores, with up to 83% of this patient population having sleep complaints.[31]

## NASAL MEDICATIONS

The standard first-line treatment of nasal obstruction is medical therapy. This treatment may include steroids or antihistamines, both intranasal and systemic and alone or in combination. There is evidence to suggest that topical medications may be beneficial in patients with nasal obstruction and concurrent sleep-related complaints. A randomized clinical trial by Craig and colleagues[32] demonstrated significant improvements in sleep quality and daytime sleepiness in patients with allergic rhinitis being treated with topical nasal steroids. The data from this study was then pooled with the results of 2 other placebo-controlled studies of intranasal corticosteroids in patients with allergic rhinitis. A significant correlation between a reduction in nasal congestion and improvement in sleep quality and sleepiness persisted.[33] Another randomized clinical trial by Kiely and colleagues[34] demonstrated significant reduction in AHI by a mean of 6.5 points; however, most patients continued to have significant OSA. Therefore, nasal steroids can improve sleep quality in this patient population and may be a useful adjunct for patients with mild OSA. This finding is in contrast to topical intranasal decongestants, which are not effective. Randomized clinical trials on the use of oxymetazoline in OSA showed no or only modest improvement in AHI scores.[35–37]

Nasal dilators that mechanically open the nasal valves have also been evaluated in patients with sleep-disordered breathing and nasal obstruction. There are 2 nasal dilators available: an externally applied Breathe Right (CNS Inc; Bloomington, MN, USA) and an internal device Nozovent (Prevancure AB, Sweden).[17] Several studies report improvement in snoring.[38–40] Of these studies, Hoijer and colleagues[39] also demonstrated improvement in OSA, with a mean decrease in the AHI by 47%, from 18.0 to 6.4. Therefore, nasal dilators may be a beneficial adjunct for patients with mild OSA. Patients who report improvement in sleep with nasal dilators may be candidates for definitive nasal valve repair.

## NASAL SURGERY

Occasionally, medical therapy is not successful in relieving nasal obstruction or a structural abnormality may be identified. In these instances, surgical intervention may be necessary. Surgical procedures to relieve nasal obstruction depend on the anatomic location of the obstruction and include, but are not limited to, septoplasty, nasal valve repair, and turbinate reduction. Additionally, endoscopic sinus surgery may have a secondary benefit of reducing inflammation in the nose, which could improve nasal resistance. There is, however, currently a dearth of data on the effect of sinus surgery on OSA.[15]

A meta-analysis published by Ishii and colleagues[41] in 2015 showed that nasal surgery improved sleep quality but not necessarily sleep apnea. A total of 225 patients from 10 studies were included in the analysis, of which 7 were prospective studies, 2 were randomized clinical trials, and 1 was retrospective in design. The meta-analysis demonstrated significant improvements in Epworth Sleepiness Scale and Respiratory Disturbance Index scores but no significant improvement in AHI. Most of the studies had relatively small sample sizes, with the largest being only 50 patients. There was also significant heterogeneity in the type of nasal surgery performed and the outcome metrics that were reported. Most of the literature compared different types of nasal surgeries, including septoplasty with or without turbinate reduction and nasal valve reconstruction. To that end, further controlled studies with a larger sample size, uniformly accepted outcome measures, and standardized nasal surgeries are needed to confirm the benefits of nasal surgery for patients with OSA.

Surgery to correct nasal obstruction may alternatively be performed with the main goal of improving tolerance of and compliance with CPAP, rather than as a cure for OSA.[42] Nakata and colleagues[43] showed an association between increased nasal resistance with poor compliance with CPAP. In their study, 12 patients with severe OSA refractory to treatment by CPAP underwent nasal surgery. Mean airway resistance measured by rhinomanometry significantly improved in all 12 patients from 0.57 Pa/cm$^3$ to 0.16 Pa/cm$^3$. Although the AHI did not change significantly, all 12 patients became tolerant to CPAP and the Epworth Sleepiness Scale score improved from 11.7 to 3.3 after surgery. Therefore, nasal surgery may facilitate treatment of patients with OSA with CPAP.

Another meta-analysis was performed to evaluate the relationship between isolated nasal surgery on therapeutic CPAP device pressures and CPAP compliance in adults with OSA.[44] Eighteen studies including 279 patients were identified. Of these, 7 studies (82 patients) reported data on CPAP pressures before and after nasal surgery, which was significantly reduced with a mean difference of 2.66 cm of water pressure. The greatest improvement was observed in patients undergoing combined septoplasty with turbinate reduction; however, subgroup analysis is hampered by the fact that only one study reported outcomes for isolated septoplasty and isolated turbinate reduction.[45]

The effect of nasal surgery on CPAP compliance and tolerance was evaluated in 11 studies (153 patients), and overall CPAP use increased postoperatively.[44] Only one study was a randomized clinical trial.[46] Subgroup analysis demonstrated that 89% (57 of 64) of patients who were not using CPAP subsequently adhered to or tolerated it after nasal surgery. It should be noted, however, that objective data were only reported in 3 studies. The investigators of this meta-analysis similarly conclude that more rigorous data in the form of controlled studies with standardized outcome measures are needed. Based on the current literature available, however, nasal surgery in patients with OSA may improve CPAP device pressures and increase CPAP use.

## SUMMARY

The nasal airway plays a significant role in breathing during sleep, and a myriad of medical and surgical interventions exist to help treat nasal obstruction in patients with concurrent sleep-disordered breathing or OSA. The current evidence suggests that these therapies can significantly improve snoring and the quality of sleep. Addressing nasal obstruction should not be viewed, however, as a means of curing OSA and should not replace the first-line treatment with CPAP. Nasal obstruction surgery can still play an important role in facilitating treatment of patients with OSA by improving tolerance and compliance with CPAP. Further controlled studies with larger sample sizes and uniformly accepted outcome measures and research methodologies are needed to fully elucidate the benefits of nasal obstruction surgery for patients with OSA.

## REFERENCES

1. Garvey JF, Pengo MF, Drakatos P, et al. Epidemiological aspects of obstructive sleep apnea. J Thorac Dis 2015;7:920–9.

2. Young T, Palta M, Dempsey J, et al. The occurrence of sleep-disordered breathing among middle-aged adults. N Engl J Med 1993;328:1230–5.

3. Newman AB, Foster G, Givelber R, et al. Progression and regression of sleep-disordered breathing with changes in weight: the Sleep Heart Health Study. Arch Intern Med 2005;165:2408–13.

4. Peppard PE, Young T, Barnet JH, et al. Increased prevalence of sleep-disordered breathing in adults. Am J Epidemiol 2013;177:1006–14.

5. Peppard PE, Young T, Palta M, et al. Prospective study of the association between sleep-disordered breathing and hypertension. N Engl J Med 2000;342: 1378–84.

6. Mooe T, Rabben T, Wiklund U, et al. Sleep-disordered breathing in men with coronary artery disease. Chest 1996;109:659–63.

7. Yaggi HK, Concato J, Kernan WN, et al. Obstructive sleep apnea as a risk factor for stroke and death. N Engl J Med 2005;353:2034–41.

8. Nieto FJ, Peppard PE, Young T, et al. Sleep-disordered breathing and cancer mortality: results from the Wisconsin Sleep Cohort Study. Am J Respir Crit Care Med 2012;186:190–4.

9. Kent BD, Grote L, Ryan S, et al. Diabetes mellitus prevalence and control in sleep-disordered breathing: the European Sleep Apnea Cohort (ESADA) study. Chest 2014;146:982–90.

10. Jackson ML, Howard ME, Barnes M. Cognition and daytime functioning in sleep-related breathing disorders. Prog Brain Res 2011;190:53–68.

11. Kakkar RK, Berry RB. Positive airway pressure treatment for obstructive sleep apnea. Chest 2007;132:1057–72.

12. Weaver TE, Grunstein RR. Adherence to continuous positive airway pressure therapy: the challenge to effective treatment. Proc Am Thorac Soc 2008;5:173–8.

13. Sawyer AM, Gooneratne NS, Marcus CL, et al. A systematic review of CPAP adherence across age groups: clinical and empiric insights for developing CPAP adherence interventions. Sleep Med Rev 2011;15:343–56.

14. Kapur VK, Auckley DH, Chowdhuri S, et al. Clinical practice guideline for diagnostic testing for adult obstructive sleep apnea: an American Academy of Sleep Medicine Clinical Practice Guideline. J Clin Sleep Med 2017;13:479–504.

15. Mickelson SA. Nasal surgery for obstructive sleep apnea syndrome. Otolaryngol Clin North Am 2016;49:1373–81.

16. Young T, Finn L, Kim H. Nasal obstruction as a risk factor for sleep-disordered breathing. The University of Wisconsin Sleep and Respiratory Research Group. J Allergy Clin Immunol 1997;99:S757–62.

17. Georgalas C. The role of the nose in snoring and obstructive sleep apnoea: an update. Eur Arch Otorhinolaryngol 2011;268:1365–73.

18. Ferris BG Jr, Mead J, Opie LH. Partitioning of respiratory flow resistance in man. J Appl Physiol 1964;19:653–8.

19. Fitzpatrick MF, Driver HS, Chatha N, et al. Partitioning of inhaled ventilation between the nasal and oral routes during sleep in normal subjects. J Appl Physiol (1985) 2003;94:883–90.

20. Park SS. Flow-regulatory function of upper airway in health and disease: a unified pathogenetic view of sleep-disordered breathing. Lung 1993;171:311–33.

21. Fitzpatrick MF, McLean H, Urton AM, et al. Effect of nasal or oral breathing route on upper airway resistance during sleep. Eur Respir J 2003;22:827–32.

22. McNicholas WT, Coffey M, Boyle T. Effects of nasal airflow on breathing during sleep in normal humans. Am Rev Respir Dis 1993;147:620–3.

23. Haight JS, Djupesland PG. Nitric oxide (NO) and obstructive sleep apnea (OSA). Sleep Breath 2003;7:53–62.

24. Suratt PM, Turner BL, Wilhoit SC. Effect of intranasal obstruction on breathing during sleep. Chest 1986;90:324–9.

25. Armengot M, Hernandez R, Miguel P, et al. Effect of total nasal obstruction on nocturnal oxygen saturation. Am J Rhinol 2008;22:325–8.

26. Friedman M, Maley A, Kelley K, et al. Impact of nasal obstruction on obstructive sleep apnea. Otolaryngol Head Neck Surg 2011;144:1000–4.

27. Turhan M, Bostanci A, Akdag M, et al. A comparison of the effects of packing or transseptal suture on polysomnographic parameters in septoplasty. Eur Arch Otorhinolaryngol 2013;270:1339–44.

28. Young T, Finn L, Palta M. Chronic nasal congestion at night is a risk factor for snoring in a population-based cohort study. Arch Intern Med 2001;161:1514–9.

29. McNicholas WT, Tarlo S, Cole P, et al. Obstructive apneas during sleep in patients with seasonal allergic rhinitis. Am Rev Respir Dis 1982;126:625–8.

30. Stuck BA, Czajkowski J, Hagner AE, et al. Changes in daytime sleepiness, quality of life, and objective sleep patterns in seasonal allergic rhinitis: a controlled clinical trial. J Allergy Clin Immunol 2004;113:663–8.

31. Kalpaklioglu AF, Kavut AB, Ekici M. Allergic and nonallergic rhinitis: the threat for obstructive sleep apnea. Ann Allergy Asthma Immunol 2009;103:20–5.

32. Craig TJ, Teets S, Lehman EB, et al. Nasal congestion secondary to allergic rhinitis as a cause of sleep disturbance and daytime fatigue and the response to topical nasal corticosteroids. J Allergy Clin Immunol 1998;101:633–7.

33. Craig TJ, Hanks CD, Fisher LH. How do topical nasal corticosteroids improve sleep and daytime somnolence in allergic rhinitis? J Allergy Clin Immunol 2005; 116:1264–6.

34. Kiely JL, Nolan P, McNicholas WT. Intranasal corticosteroid therapy for obstructive sleep apnoea in patients with co-existing rhinitis. Thorax 2004;59:50–5.

35. Kerr P, Millar T, Buckle P, et al. The importance of nasal resistance in obstructive sleep apnea syndrome. J Otolaryngol 1992;21:189–95.

36. McLean HA, Urton AM, Driver HS, et al. Effect of treating severe nasal obstruction on the severity of obstructive sleep apnoea. Eur Respir J 2005;25:521–7.

37. Clarenbach CF, Kohler M, Senn O, et al. Does nasal decongestion improve obstructive sleep apnea? J Sleep Res 2008;17:444–9.

38. Petruson B. Snoring can be reduced when the nasal airflow is increased by the nasal dilator Nozovent. Arch Otolaryngol Head Neck Surg 1990;116:462–4.

39. Hoijer U, Ejnell H, Hedner J, et al. The effects of nasal dilation on snoring and obstructive sleep apnea. Arch Otolaryngol Head Neck Surg 1992;118:281–4.

40. Pevernagie D, Hamans E, Van Cauwenberge P, et al. External nasal dilation reduces snoring in chronic rhinitis patients: a randomized controlled trial. Eur Respir J 2000;15:996–1000.

41. Ishii L, Roxbury C, Godoy A, et al. Does nasal surgery improve OSA in patients with nasal obstruction and OSA? A meta-analysis. Otolaryngol Head Neck Surg 2015;153:326–33.

42. Poirier J, George C, Rotenberg B. The effect of nasal surgery on nasal continuous positive airway pressure compliance. Laryngoscope 2014;124:317–9.

43. Nakata S, Noda A, Yagi H, et al. Nasal resistance for determinant factor of nasal surgery in CPAP failure patients with obstructive sleep apnea syndrome. Rhinology 2005;43:296–9.

44. Camacho M, Riaz M, Capasso R, et al. The effect of nasal surgery on continuous positive airway pressure device use and therapeutic treatment pressures: a systematic review and meta-analysis. Sleep 2015;38:279–86.

45. Zonato AI, Bittencourt LR, Martinho FL, et al. Upper airway surgery: the effect on nasal continuous positive airway pressure titration on obstructive sleep apnea patients. Eur Arch Otorhinolaryngol 2006;263:481–6.

46. Powell NB, Zonato AI, Weaver EM, et al. Radiofrequency treatment of turbinate hypertrophy in subjects using continuous positive airway pressure: a randomized, double-blind, placebo-controlled clinical pilot trial. Laryngoscope 2001; 111:1783–90.

# Moving?

## Make sure your subscription moves with you!

To notify us of your new address, find your **Clinics Account Number** (located on your mailing label above your name), and contact customer service at:

**Email: journalscustomerservice-usa@elsevier.com**

**800-654-2452** (subscribers in the U.S. & Canada)
**314-447-8871** (subscribers outside of the U.S. & Canada)

**Fax number: 314-447-8029**

**Elsevier Health Sciences Division**
**Subscription Customer Service**
**3251 Riverport Lane**
**Maryland Heights, MO 63043**

*To ensure uninterrupted delivery of your subscription, please notify us at least 4 weeks in advance of move.